Essential Oils and Aromatherapy:

The Reference guide of Ancient Medicine for Natural Remedies, Young Living and Weight Loss...for You and Your Dog

Table of Contents

L'indice è vuoto perché non stai utilizzando gli stili paragrafo che hai scelto di visualizzarvi.

© Copyright 2018 by Axe Dr Raskin- All rights reserved.

The following eBook is reproduced below with the goal of providing information that is as accurate and reliable as possible. Regardless, purchasing this eBook can be seen as consent to the fact that both the publisher and the author of this book are in no way experts on the topics discussed within and that any recommendations or suggestions that are made herein are for entertainment purposes only. Professionals should be consulted as needed prior to undertaking any of the action endorsed herein.

This declaration is deemed fair and valid by both the American Bar Association and the Committee of Publishers Association and is legally binding throughout the United States.

Furthermore, the transmission, duplication, or reproduction of any of the following work including specific information will be considered an illegal act irrespective of if it is done electronically or in print. This extends to creating a secondary or tertiary copy of the work or a recorded copy and is only allowed with the express written consent from the Publisher. All additional right reserved.

The information in the following pages is broadly considered a truthful and accurate account of facts and as such, any inattention, use, or misuse of the information in question by the reader will render any resulting actions solely under their purview. There are no scenarios in which the publisher or the original author of this work can be in any fashion deemed liable for any hardship or damages that may befall them after undertaking information described herein.

Additionally, the information in the following pages is intended only for informational purposes and should thus be thought of as universal. As befitting its nature, it is presented without assurance regarding its prolonged validity or interim quality. Trademarks that are mentioned are done without written consent and can in no way be considered an endorsement from the trademark holder.

Introduction

Essential oils are extracted from several different methods that were first created by the Egyptians around the 1500 BC. They are used to help you with herbal alternative medicines that can alleviate as well as eliminate your ailments. Many people are suffering from ailments that have no cure from modern medicine. They then turn to alternative remedies and these are helping lead them to Essential Oils. Since Essential Oils are the essence of the plant and plants are nature's own medicine, it does not surprise me that they have been used to heal, perfume, embalm, and deodorize for centuries.

This book will help you understand the past of how Essential Oils have been used and what to expect from them when you start developing your own blends. Now that you have purchased this *Essential Oils and Aromatherapy* book you will be one step ahead with a few basic pieces of knowledge that will help you build your aromatherapy arsenal within your home starting with Lavender, Cedarwood, Sandalwood, Tea Tree oil, and many others.

There are a few basic oils that you can start with and then there are more advanced and costly oils that can be used in some special recipes. When starting out, you want to start with the more affordable options and then advance yourself slowly so that you do not jump too far into the Essential Oil industry and buy that $400 rose oil.

Chapter 1: What are essential oils?

Essential Oils are often being thought of, as the oil of a plant, but they are much more than that. To cultivate the oil of a plant you have to go through a process of distillation, enfleurage, expression, solvents, as well as carbon dioxide. This process uses the plants as a way to extract the essence of them into what is called an essential oil. Every single living plant on this planet has an essence that can be extracted through a process of either distillation, expression, enfleurage, and solvents, which are the most common types of extraction methods. Scientists have been working on new methods of extraction that utilizes the compounds found in carbon dioxide.

To distill oils, you must first pick the flowers and plant leaves from the subject and then place them in a position that allows them to hang over water which is boiling. The steam is then used to pull the essence from the plant's stems, flowers, and leaves. Once the steam rises it is pushed through a vessel that allows it to travel, while rapidly cooling to another holding cell. This rapid cooling will allow it to condense into a water form; the oil of the plant will then separate itself from the water and would be easy to scoop out of the water.

This process then allows the scientists to collect the essence of the plant, while also leaving behind the aromatics that many aroma-therapists will collect and are highly seeking. These aromatics are called hydrosols. Not all plants are left with a hydrosol, but many are. Hydrosols are the aromatics that are used in makeup and moisturizers for skin.

The process of using enfleurage, which is an outdated process that is not used often other than in France, can be accomplished by a complicated method. Not only is the method complicated, but it is quite expensive as well. By placing blossoms on a warm flat piece of fat, the oils from the plant will be absorbed into the fat. After the oil has incorporated fully into the fat, those flowers are tossed, and the scientists will replace the flowers with more healthy flowers. In the past, animal lard and fat was being used. This process is done several times in order to infuse the fat with the fragrant aromas of the flowers. Once this process is completed, the fat is then separated by using a process of solvents which allows for the oil to be removed.

The process by which expression is used would be accomplished by using the flesh of plants, skins, as well as the seeds. This process is similar to what you would find the olive oil makers use to make the olive oil that we use for cooking. By using the peels of citrus fruits, which include oranges, limes, grapefruits, lemons, and other citrus from which you are able to peel off the skin and then press the oil out of them, one can produce very potent essential oils. So be careful with these citrus type oils. They will be stronger and have more potency to them.

When using solvents to extract essential oils it is best to not use the ones based on a chemical compound. This can leave a slight trace of solvent chemicals which many aromatherapists believe can damage the potency and purity of the essential oil. Although it is believed that the solvent is no longer remaining once the oil is produced, many aromatherapists prefer to stay away from this type of extraction method. This process is accomplished by placing the plant in the solvent and dissolving it in hexane, methylene of chlorure, and benzene. This solvent has a lower boiling point; it is then evaporated so that none is remaining when the oils are ready. This can be accomplished through a machine that will use a process similar to centrifugal force or vacuuming out the essential oil.

Once the oil is removed, it is called an absolute. There are other methods for this process such as paraffin wax, which will not completely evaporate off the solvents. This leaves behind some paraffin which can cause your base essential oil to become a solid which makes it a concrete, instead of an absolute. Once the process of the solvent is evaporated and then subsequently cooled and recaptured into a liquid the process is much more expensive. This is mostly reserved for the oils that are much costlier and have no distillation ability. This works best for vanilla and jasmine, as well as rose. This helps the essential oil to be less expensive, only slightly, when extracted in this process.

Carbon dioxide has been experimented with recently for a new process of extraction. However, the method is expensive; it is quite an interesting process. This process helps produce an aromatic essential oil that smells similar to the actual plant itself.

By producing an essential oil through any one of these methods you are influencing the quality as well as the concentration level by which the levels are. Although essential oils are a beneficial treatment device for many of our ailments they can be misused and cause potential threats to your system if not used properly. In the next few chapters, I will go over the details that will make it possible for you to utilize Essential Oils in your healthcare, home cleaning, and general daily activities. Essential Oils are a wonderful way to add aromatic plant-based natural healing energies into your life as well as a great way to clean your home.

Chapter 2: History of the Use of Essential Oils in Aromatherapy

For thousands of years, humans have been searching for a way to cure their ailments. They have practiced herbalism, chemistry, and even metaphysical ways to heal. Many of the ways that they have used to alleviate their symptoms did not always work out. Some created more complications; some were simply too delusional to work. Nevertheless, one that has always stuck around is the use of essential oils.

The use of essential oils has documented proof that dates back all the way to before the Ancient Egyptians. As early as 3000 B.C., essential oils have been showing up in medicinal records and historical documents. However, the earliest contributions within the historical text were specific to the Chinese region—later came the use by Egyptians, Romans, and many other cultures. If you look even further back, you will find a few references to Ayurvedic use from India. In the early 2000 B.C., the Egyptians started to find multiple uses for essential oils. This included enhancement to spiritual practices, bathing and beauty products, and even benefits that provide a medicinal aspect. With a strong passion for beauty and being beautiful, the Egyptians developed treatment programs and care regimes that would help them look their best at all times. It was a standard practice for Egyptians, including Cleopatra, to use the fatty oils, essential oils, and even salts or clays to take care of their hygiene and skin care needs. They would collect salt and clay from the Dead Sea—which is located within Egypt—and even Marc Anthony gifted these to Cleopatra with such luxuries.

The aromatic scents that come from essential oils have also found its way into the perfume industry. In history, you will find that queens, kings, pharaohs, priests, and even doctors have all used essential oils in some way. The fact that essential oils are so versatile can clearly show the major benefits that can be gained by learning all you can about their uses and capabilities within the human mind, body, and spirit.

If we examine closely how essential oils first began gaining popularity within the various cultures, then you will be able to have a strong understanding of the versatility of essential oils—not only in history but also in your own life.

Dordogne Region Within France

Pieces of evidence within the cave drawings suggest the use of essential oils as early as 18,000 B.C.E. This carbon dating has been scientifically proven and recorded.

Egypt

The recorded history of essential oil use within the Egyptian culture can be found as early as 4500 B.C.E. Since the Egyptians developed a method of cosmetology that many still practice today, it is no surprise to find that they were using essential oils for everything, from cosmetics to embalming. Although many people within Egyptian history utilized essential oils for various methods and uses, at the most powerful point in Egyptian history, only priests were allowed to possess these oils. Within the Egyptian practices, they designated a specific fragrance for each one of the deities that they worshipped. They would then use that oil to anoint the statues of the deities for religious celebration and offerings.

China's Essential Oil Culture

China has recordings of essential oil usage that dates all the way back to 2697 B.C.E. This time period took place during the Huang Ti Dynasty, which was run by the Yellow Emperor who is legendary in his own right. At the height of his power he penned the book "The Yellow Emperor Book of Internal Medicine." This book is full of medicinal recipes that have shown to be beneficial to the human body, mind, and spirit.

They contain some of the first recordings of Eastern Medicine.

India's Essential Oil Culture

The culture in the Indies that has been supporting the use of essential oils over the past 3000 years by a method called Ayur Veda. This process is developed to help people utilize healing potions as well as Vedic nutrition that includes over 700 essential oil substance such as Myrrh, Ginger, Sandalwood and many more. When the Bubonic Plaque was threatening life in every country, Ayur Veda was utilized, quite successfully to replace antibiotics that were ineffective against the disease. The Indians developed spiritual practices around the use of essential oils as well which were integral in the role of the philosophy behind Ayurvedic medicine.

Greece

Greeks have been using essential oils since 500 B.C.E to help with medicinal uses. They developed their methods through the written records that came from the Egyptians and their extensive knowledge of essential oils and their uses. Hypocrites, the father of medicine, penned a written document that shows the uses and effects of over 300 medicinal plants.

Hypocrites also used the practice of Ayurvedic in their essential oil medicinal methods. He showed a great connection between the Greeks and the Egyptian and Indian practices. The Greek soldiers experienced this connection when traveling with Alexander the Great during his travels. The development of Ayur Veda was found to be a balancing practice that brought harmony to their medical practices. This helped them mingle the traditions together developing a method that worked for them.

One of Hypocrites practices that he wrote about within his journals was, a bath infused with essential oils and then a massage infused with essential oils was a daily necessity for perfect health. Through his teachings and the literature that was left behind by him and his students, he left us with the most important message about medicine. The Doctors purpose should be awakening the energies for natural healing within in your own body. This helped develop the Hippocratic Oath that is taken upon receiving their license for all Doctors.

Rome's Essential Oil Culture

Essential oils were used to lavishly cover the Romans bodies with the perfumed oils, as well as their clothes and even bedding. They believed in having a mass amount of fragrance enveloping them at all times. They also used essential oils to massage their partners and within their baths. They brought the books written by Hypocrites and Galen when fleeing the country during the fall of the Roman Empire. Later on, these texts were used to help the Persians, and Arabic's learn of the medicinal uses for essential oils, by being translated into the appropriate language.

Persian Essential Oil Culture

One of the youngest Physicians was from Persia. His name was Ali-Ibn Sana and he lived in 980-1037 A.D. He gained his doctoral at 12 and authored several books that detailed the medicinal benefits of plants on the human body. He also was the first person to be credited with documented proof and methods for distillation of essential oils. The methods that Ali-Ibn Sana developed and wrote about are still used today.

Europe's Essential Oil Culture

The knights and crusaders who traveled to the Middle East and Western Europe have been tasked with the responsibility to pass on their knowledge base for the medicinal use of herbs. These knights would carry fragrances with them as they traveled and pass on the details of distillation. They believed that Pine and Frankincense would ward off evil spirits, so they burned these in the streets, this took place during the Bubonic Plaque that threatened lives during the 14th Century. There are written records that show that this process helped to lower the number of deaths in those areas.

This led to the 1653 publication of "The Complete Herbal" which was written by Nicholas Culpepper. This book still stands as one of the most valuable resources for those wishing to practice the use of medicinal herbs. In this book, you will find several ailments and conditions along with remedies that will help still today.

Rene-Maurice Gattefosse, who was a French chemist, developed and coined the term Aromatherapy, which details the proper uses of essential oils and how they can help you. He learned the hard way of how beneficial essential oils are by getting burned in a lab fire and utilizing Lavender oil to heal his burns.

Since there is such an extensive history of essential oils and their uses for medicinal benefits, it's hard to believe that so many people are still not educated on the proper use and benefits. This book is designed to provide those who are lacking in the educational background in essential oils, all the information they need to utilize such a wonderful and extensively used product for their health and well-being.

This chapter discussed the History of essential oils. You will learn about each country roll in the development of what is called Aromatherapy in today's Essential oil world. You will also learn some specific points in history that give credit to the benefits of essential oils when dealing with medical issues and concerns. Once you delve deep into this chapter you will begin to see the advantages that essential oils bring to your life.

Next, you will jump to chapter 2 and learn all the ways that essential oils can influence your weight loss journey. I will discuss the oils that are specific to weight loss and how they help you increase your chances of weight loss success. as well as the specific oils that will need to be incorporated into your lifestyle to begin losing weight.

Chapter 3: How can they be used as an alternative to modern medicine?

If you are reading this book, then I am sure you have heard of all the wonderful benefits that are received from the use of Essential Oils in your daily life. Not only do they provide for a cleaner fresher air system within your home, but they are known to alleviate and often times eliminate common ailments that are found within women, men, and children throughout life.

The use of Essential Oils started all the way back in Ancient Egypt back before the invention of modern medicine. In ancient Egypt, the kings and queens believed that the aromatic essences of the plants were a gift to everyone, even slaves were awarded or given essential oils for perfumes, healing potentials, and other uses. In fact, the original embalming solution was created with essential oils.

Since the history of Essential Oils is a twisting and winding labyrinth of herbal medicine and magical practices through all cultures, it is best to start with the Egyptians and how they made way for the use of Essential Oils in all aspects of your life, including death. The use of Essential Oils is not only stemmed in ailment and medicine, but also in enhancement of life. Since many cultures hold believes around the magic of the plant it is only natural that the world would come to the conclusion that Essential Oils are beneficial and enhance our life as well as health. With the use of rituals, cooking, and medicine in the history of every culture, knowing what Essential Oils are best for you is as simple as picking up a book, such as this one.

The amazing thing about Essential Oils and incense is that they were even addressed within the religious text as a gift or therapeutic practice used among even the holiest of believers. To be anointed by a priest with oils that are fragrant, or perfumes was a rite of passage for many religious practices as well as universal for most religious sects. It is believed that using an incense dowsed in Essential Oils is a great way to connect with the spiritual world.

Due to the long-time written history of the use of Essential Oils, such as the Ebers Papyrus dating back to 1500 BC in Egypt, you are able to obtain an in-depth knowledge and training in Essential Oils form just about any reputable source, like this one. I have filled this book with several helpful tips and recipes that will help you to incorporate

Essential Oils into your health routine, living environment, and enhancing of life practices, as well as religious usage.

How can you utilize Essential Oils for medicinal purposes?

Essential Oils have been used by herbal practitioners for over 1000-6000 years, depending on the cultural background and usage. The uses of Essential Oils are widespread among many different ailments, as well as enhancement of life. The ancient Egyptians used Cinnamon, Clove, Myrrh, Nutmeg, and Cedarwood oil to embalm the dead. Megallus, the Greek perfumer, created a Myrrh and fat-based oil for anti-inflammatory as well as skin healing for wounds. In the 12th century the Abbess of Germany, known as Hildegard, harvested and distilled his own Lavender for the properties that it provided with medicinal use.

By using the inhalation method, you can begin to see changes in your ailments. When you use a diffuser the process of heating water and then vaporizing the oils within that water creates a steam bath that can alleviate many airborne pathogens as well as enhance your mental health and clear out germs in your environment. Not only is there a pleasant aroma that emits from the diffuser, but they are able to provide respiratory aids with certain oils used, as well as a decongestion aid, and even psychological aids.

By inhaling your oils in the steam bath, you are able to inhale the aromatic medicine and stimulate the olfactory which is located in the brain and connects your brain with the aromas that are coming in through your mouth and nose. Once these molecules enter your olfactory sensors, they will pass to the lungs and then subsequently to the rest of the body.

On top of the inhalation process, there is also a topical process which can be utilized through the use of oils for massage, as well as skin care, and baths. By applying oil to the muscles and other painful regions you can massage the oils into the tissue and boost the circulation which helps to absorb the medicinal properties of the Essential Oils. There is a long-time belief that locations with sweat glands or follicles for hair around the palms and head can absorb more oil and in a more effective manner.

There is a process of dilution that must be done prior to using Essential Oils on your skin, so be mindful of the oils that you are applying and make sure that you apply them in the proper way. Most of the oils will need to be diluted to a certain percentage based on the concentration level they are. These details will be discussed a bit later in this book with each recipe, however, I wanted to touch on the details a bit here.

There are a few carrier oils that can be used to dilute the Essential Oils and it is mostly based on purpose, as well as personal preference. If you have a high allergy probability, then you should check for allergic reaction prior to using them.

Knowing the profiles of your oils can determine the types of uses they would be good for in a medicinal way. For instance, tea tree oil is great for use with acne, infections that are fungal based, lice, athletes foot, scabies, ringworm, and other microbial germs. But that is not all you can do with Tea Tree oil. In fact, tea tree oils are so effective at so many different things that many people, including myself, make it a staple in their household. What other remedy do you know that can cure ear infections, toothache, ringworm, lice, insect bites, boils, infections within the nose or mouth, herpes labialis, scabies, athlete's foot, acne as well as treat a cough, pulmonary inflammation, and clean your home of germs? There are a few things to consider before using tea tree oil though. These are related to pregnancy and breastfeeding mothers. You should never apply or use tea tree oil while breastfeeding or pregnant and never swallow or ingest tea tree oil since it is toxic. For young boys, you should avoid using tea tree oil with lavender since it will possibly affect their hormones and disrupt the normal process they undergo during puberty.

Another very popular medicinal use for Essential Oils is the use of lavender oil. Although many people talk about Lavender Oil, do they really know the full range of benefits that Lavender Oil can provide? Probably, Not. So, getting to know the oils you use and the benefits from using them is key to effectively use them for an effective medicinal purpose. In ancient Egypt, the use of Lavender Oil provided a way to mummify the deceased loved ones. Many of the tomb archeologists have stated that the scent of lavender was detected for over 3000 years within the tombs of the Pharaohs and Kings. It is also a great use for antibacterial benefits, as well as digestive system types of diseases and rheumatoid arthritis. The benefits of Lavender Oil can be seen in the benefits it provides for the alleviation of headaches, heal some burns, improve your sleep, reduce anxiety and stress that is emotionally charged, restore the skin from complexion issues and then reduce the acne that is associated with the complexion issue, relieve pain for arthritic joints, and protect from diabetes type symptoms. It is gentle enough for a direct application which makes it a great oil to have in your go-to kit for medicinal purposes.

Another great oil with some wonderful medicinal benefits is Peppermint Oil. Peppermint is a cross breed between water mint and spearmint, which can be cultivated form North America and Europe. Many chefs or bakers will use peppermint oil in their baking and cook for flavor as well as in beverages for a wonderful twist. You can also find it applied in soaps and cosmetics for a wonderful cooling effect. It is great as a dietary supplement along with health benefits through topical use and ointments. It is widely known that the use of peppermint oil is great for those who suffer from irritable bowel syndrome. Since it aids with digestion of your food and the prevention of stomach spasms within your GI tract you can avoid endoscopy or barium enema. When used for a topical relief of headaches and nipples that are cracked from the breastfeeding practice it is quite soothing. However, you must be aware of the side effects that have been reported such as, interaction with specific medications, and heartburn.

These are just a few of the oils that can provide relief for so many medical ailments. With the large and vast variety of oils on the market, it would be difficult to get the complete picture of their use in this one chapter. But I can give you a basic idea that will help you get started on your Essential Oil herbal path. In the next chapter, I will go over several easy to follow recipes with dilution steps and proper preparation methods for several ailments that could be affecting your family.

Chapter 4: Essence Oils Basics

There are several oils that make the list of necessary purchases when starting out with essence oils. Below, I will include all the details that you will need to know about those oils and what makes them so special. This is not a comprehensive list of oils since there are over 200 oils, but this is a beginners list that will bring you on the journey of natural healing and a healthy lifestyle.

Profiles for Medicinal Use

Bergamot

Bergamot is a citrus-based scent and it helps with the alleviation of:
- Nervous Tension
- Nervous System Balances
- Disinfection
- Uplifting Mood
- Anxiety Reduction
- Stress Reduction

Cajeput

Cajeput is a camphor-based scent and it helps with the alleviation of:
- Insect Repellant
- Helps with Restful Sleep
- Congestion Break Up

- Warms the Inside of Your Body
- Calming Effect
- Helps Relax Those Muscles That Get Tight
- Alleviates Muscle Pains and Ache
- Helps with Breathing by Using Vapors
- Disinfectant

Clary Sage

Clary Sage is a spicy and sweet-based scent and it helps with the alleviation of:

- Communication Encouragement
- Hormone Balancing with Estrogen
- Sleep Aid
- Aphrodisiac
- Digestive Aid
- Pain Reducer
- Calming
- Stress Reduction
- Tension Relief

Chamomile

Chamomile is a musk-based scent and it helps with the alleviation of:

- Insect Bite Soother
- Calming
- Sleep Aid
- Appetite Improver
- Skin Healer
- Digestive Aid

- Inflammation Reduction
- Pain Reducer
- Stress Reduction
- Tension Relief

Clove

Clove is a hot and spicy-based scent and it helps with the alleviation of:

- Insect Repellant
- Uplifts Moods
- Fatigue Reducer
- Aphrodisiac
- Digestion Aid
- Disinfectant
- Breathing Aid with Vapors
- Pain Reducer
- Mental Clarity Improvement
- Memory Aid

Eucalyptus

Eucalyptus is camphor-like with a fresh-based scent and it helps with the alleviation of:

- Insect Repellant
- Breathing Aid with Vapors
- Body Cooling
- Pain Reducer
- Congestion Reduction
- Refreshing
- Inflammation Reducer

- Disinfectant

Grapefruit

Grapefruit scent is citrus-based, and it helps with the alleviation of:
- Purifies the Body
- Cellulite Reduction of Deposits
- Physical Strength Is Increased
- Cooling Effect on the Body
- Uplifting the Mood
- Refreshing
- Energizing
- Mental Clarity Is Improved
- Memory Is Improved
- Fatigue Is Relieved

Geranium

Geranium scent is rose-based, and it helps with the alleviation of:
- Insect Repellant
- Itchy Skin Soother
- Pain Reducer
- Stress Reduction
- Tension Relief
- Stimulating in Doses That Are Large
- Uplifting of Your Mood
- Inflammation Reduction
- Cellulite Reduction of Deposits
- Bleeding Aid for Injuries

- Communication Encouragement
- Calming in Doses That Are Small

Lemongrass

Lemongrass' scent is a lemon-based and it helps with the alleviation of:

- Insect Repellant
- Digestion Aid
- Breathing Aid with Vapors
- Weak Connective Tissues Are Contracted
- Lactation Stimulation
- Inflammation Reduction
- Calming
- Uplifting Mood
- Nervous System Balances Out
- Skin Is Toned
- Disinfection

Cedarwood

Cedarwood scent is woody-based and it helps with the alleviation of:

- Insect Repellant
- Pain Reducer
- Meditation Assistant
- Calming
- Anxiety Reducer
- Tension Reliever
- Sleep Aid
- Breathing Aid with Vapors

Jasmine

Jasmine is a sweet floral-based scent and it helps with the alleviation of:
- Aphrodisiac
- Uplifting Mood

Myrrh

Myrrh is a bitter-based scent and it helps with the alleviation of:
- Skin Is Healed
- Meditation Assistant
- Uplifting Mood
- Inflammation Relief

Lavender

Lavender is a clean and fresh-based scent and it helps with the alleviation of:
- Insect Repellant
- Skin Is Healed
- Disinfectant
- Digestion Improvement
- Breathing Improves with Vapors
- Congestion Will Break Up
- Sleep Will Improve
- Inflammation Reduction
- Uplifting Mood
- Tight Muscles Relax
- Stress Is Reduced

- Tension Is Relieved
- Stimulating in Larger Doses
- Calming in Smaller Doses
- Mood Swings Are Balanced
- Purifies the Body
- Insect Bites Are Soothed
- Pain Relief

Frankincense

Frankincense is camphor-like and woody-based scent and it helps with the alleviation of:
- Skin Rejuvenator
- Wrinkle Reducer
- Inflammation Reduction
- Communication Enhancer
- Sleep Aid
- Mediation Assistant
- Calming

Lemon

Lemon is a lemony-based scent and it helps with the alleviation of:
- Insect Bites Are Soothed
- Bleeding from Injuries Is Stopped
- Refreshing
- Disinfectant
- Body Is Purified
- Mental Clarity Is Improved
- Memory Is Improved

- Uplifting the Mood
- Fatigue Is Relieved
- Nervous System Is Balanced
- Energizing
- Calming
- Balancing
- Cooling Effect on the Body
- Cellulite Deposits Are Reduced

Neroli

Neroli is a sweet floral-based scent and it helps with the alleviation of:

- Uplifting Mood
- Sleep Aid
- Nervous Tension Relief

Orange

Orange is a sweet orange-based scent and it helps with the alleviation of:

- Purifies the Body
- Uplifting Mood
- Cools the Body
- Sleep Improvement
- Calming
- Stress Reduction

Patchouli

Patchouli is a musk-based scent and it helps with the alleviation of:

- Insect Repellant
- Disinfectant
- Uplifting Mood
- Aphrodisiac
- Stimulates the Nerves
- Skin Rejuvenating

Peppermint

Peppermint is a strong minty-based scent and it helps with the alleviation of:

- Insect Repellant
- Relieves and Soothes Skin That Is Itchy
- Mental Clarity Improvement
- Memory Improvement
- Lactation Reduction
- Appetite Improvement
- Inflammation Reducers
- Digestion Improvement
- Refreshing
- Aphrodisiac
- Stimulates the Nerves
- Breathing Improvement with Vapors
- Congestion Improvement
- Fatigue Relief
- Pain Reduction
- Cools the Body Down
- Uplifting Moods
- Energizing

Rosemary

Rosemary is a camphor-based strong scent and it helps with the alleviation of:
- Insect Repellant
- Cellulite Deposit Reduction
- Disinfectant
- Energizing
- Tight Muscles Reduced
- Pain Reduction
- Stimulates the Nerves
- Digestion Improvement
- Mental Clarity Improvement
- Memory Improvement
- Purifies the Body
- Fatigue Relief
- Uplifting Moods

Sandalwood

Sandalwood is a woody-based scent and it helps with the alleviation of:
- Skin Healing
- Uplifting Mood
- Aphrodisiac
- Meditation Assistant
- Calming
- Stress Reduction
- Sleep Improvement

Sage

Sage is a spicy-based scent and it helps with the alleviation of:
- Disinfectant
- Pain Reducer
- Lactation Reducer
- Perspiration Reducer
- Purifies the Body

Palmarosa

Palmarosa is a sweet-based scent and it helps with the alleviation of:
- Healing
- Moisturizing
- Regenerating
- Inflammation Reduction
- Pain Reducer
- Warms the Body
- Tight Muscles Relieved
- Uplifting Mood

Tea Tree

Tea Tree is a camphor-like-based scent and it helps with the alleviation of:
- Skin Healing
- Breathing Improvement with Vapors
- Pain Reduction
- Disinfectant

Thyme

Thyme is a hot and spicy-based scent and it helps with the alleviation of:

- Insect Repellant
- Purifies the Body
- Perspiration Increase
- Appetite Improvement
- Cellulite Deposits Reduction
- Disinfectant
- Mental Clarity Improvement
- Memory Improvement
- Digestion Improvement
- Breathing Improvement with Vapors
- Inflammation Reduction
- Congestion Improvement
- Physical Strength Advancement
- Uplifting Moods
- Aphrodisiac
- Pain Reduction
- Warms the Body
- Tight Muscles Reduced

This is just a few of the essential oils that you can use for the recipes further along in this book. Although this is not a comprehensive bible of essential oils, it is a great place to get started along your journey.

Application Methods

The application methods for essential oils are pretty easy to remember. When applying oil to a sore or injured part, you simply apply it directly to the injured or sore location. When using an aromatic effect, you will be able to use a diffuser or an inhaler. You can also use the neti pot. In applying, to have a full body effect, you can apply to several points on your body.

These include:
- Temples
- Behind the ears
- On the back of your neck
- Under your arms on your feet
- Wrists
- Forehead

All of these application methods can be utilized depending on the effect that you are trying to receive. Men, women, and children are all able to handle essence oils depending on the type of oil it is and the health conditions that they are dealing with.

Blending Properly

The proper blending technique is needed to maintain a pure aromatherapy blend. In order to blend oils, you will need to start with a glass container or dram to blend them in.

Next, you will need to apply the oil or oils that you are using the most drops from. This allows you to add in the highest dosage to the lowest dosage with the oils. Once the oils are all applied to the dram or container, you should place the lid on the container or dram and roll the bottle between your palms. Next, using your first finger and thumb, flip the bottle upside down and then right side up. This helps to incorporate the oils together. You can also start by twirling the oils in the bottle to ensure that all the oil is located at the bottom of the dram or container.

After blending the oils properly, you will need to then pour in any carrier oil that you are using. Remember, every single oil should be used with precaution and most of them require a blending effect with carrier oils. There are several carrier oils that you can use. Below is a list of the most common ones.

- Almond
- Coconut
- Olive
- Grapeseed
- Macadamia
- Peach Kernel
- Apricot Kernel
- Hazelnut
- Camellia
- Wheat Germ
- Rosehip
- Borage

- Carrot
- Evening Primrose
- Avocado
- Jojoba
- And several others

Precautions to Take

There are several precautions that you will need to take when using oils on women, men, and children, as well as pets.

Women

Pregnant women should abstain from using essence oils. Although there are a few that are found for pregnancy and lactation, it is best to avoid since the unborn could be allergic and it could potentially harm them.

The ones that are safe in small and ridiculously small amounts:
- Cardamom
- Geranium
- Coriander
- Ginger
- Lavender
- Grapefruit
- Spearmint
- Petitgrain
- Ylang-Ylang
- Melissa
- Palmarosa

- Mandarin
- Lime
- Lemongrass
- Lavender
- Lemon
- Neroli

Precautions and Procedures to Follow

Those with lots of allergic reactions should take precautions to determine if they are allergic to any of the essential oils. To test your allergic reaction, take these steps:
- Rub your chest with a carrier oil
- Wait 12 hours
- Examine for red or itchy skin

If there is no irritation, then you can start to test essence oils:
- Add 1 drop of any essential oil you wish to try within 15 drops of the carrier oil.
- If there is no reaction after the oil has sat on your skin for 12 hours, then you will be safe.

Another thing to remember is that oils do not need to be applied directly to these areas:
- The eyes
- The lips
- The genitals
- Or any other sensitive area prior to testing

If you get oil in your eyes, it is best to try to flush it with water or use sweet almond oil and place a drop into the eye to neutralize the oil.

Alcohol is not a great combination when using essential oils; however, a glass of wine at dinner is perfectly acceptable. Avoid sunlight exposure when you directly applied citrus since this can cause the skin to burn with the exposure. These skins can be irritating to your skin so take precautions and use sparingly:

- Clove
- Lemongrass
- Cinnamon
- Mandarin
- Melissa
- Lemon
- Grapefruit
- Peppermint
- Orange
- Spearmint
- Black Pepper

If you suffer from sensitive skin, then you should apply these oils in a bath, for hands, body, and feet, at half strength. They should not be used if you are taking medication that could be altered by the oils.

All essential oils need to be stored properly and high above a child's reach. If oils are stored in light and oxygenated oils, they will begin to deteriorate. Use a dark and cool environment for storage. Refrigerating them will slow down the rate of spoilage. All bottles need to be closed tightly. This prevents evaporating and oxidizing. Handle your oils carefully so that you do not ruin furniture and wood finish. The lifespan of a refined essence oil is one year whilst unrefined would be shorter in lifespan. Therefore, store them in the fridge once opened to extend their lifespan. Most oils will live for 1 to 2 years when stored properly. Citrus only stays alive for 6 to 9 months depending on storage and usage.

Every person is on some form of medication for an ailment. Before starting an essence oil regimen, make sure the oils will not interfere with the ailments that you have. For instance, low blood pressure patients and heart patients should not use grapefruit oil. Babies should not use tea tree oil or anything that is camphor based.

Chapter 5: The Best Location to Purchase Your Oils for Your Home Health Care Needs and What to Look for When Buying Them

There are many companies that provide essence oils for purchasing, however, how do you know if they are the perfect company for you? First, you need to examine how pure and authentic the oils are. This can be done in several ways. To test the oils from a company, you should purchase a sample of some of the oils that you wish to purchase. Then test them in the white cardstock test.

The White Cardstock Tests

Choose the oil that you wish to use and drip one drop on the cardstock. After 48 hours, the oil should be evaporated, leaving no trace, smell, or color unless it is citrus oil that is colored. This will show the purity of the oil and that it has not been altered.

The Water Tests

Choose the oil that you wish to use. Drip it into the water. If it turns milky or changes the color of the water, then it has been altered.

Check the Pricing

If the pricing is all too similar in range or is much lower than other companies, then they are not selling pure, authentic oils. However, this works in reverse as well. If the pricing is outrageously higher than reputable companies, then they are not selling pure, authentic oils as well, and they are using the pricing to fake the quality of the product. If you see rose oil for ½-ounce or 1-ounce increments and it is affordable, then steer clear. The only ones sold in .5 ml, or .10 ml containers and a .5 ml container is about $295.

A few reputable companies that have never had a controversial situation over their products or methods would be:

- Mountain Rose Herb

    www.mountainroseherb.com

- Plant Therapy

    www.planttherapy.com

- Florihana

www.florihana.com

- Fragrant Earth

    www.fragrant-earth.com

- Essence Aura Aromatherapy

    www.essentialaura.com

    www.organicfair.com

Chapter 6: How Essential Oils Can Influence Your Weight Loss Goals

Essential oils have been instrumental in helping people heal from multiple different ailments, and in this book, I will discuss the benefits that you will find when utilizing essential oils for losing weight.

Many people suffer having difficulty in achieving weight loss. They spend thousands of dollars a month on fad diets and exercise programs that they never use. They beg and plead with God and ask for the easy way to lose weight. Many people may actually try to lose weight, but most will simply complain that it is too hard or reason out that altering their portions and how much they eat per day will only make them hungrier. This becomes an endless cycle of wanting a change but never actually accomplishing it. After years of trying to lose weight without actually putting the effort out, they will seek medical intervention and get on diet pills or have gastric bypass surgery.

However, these are only a temporary fix, since the habits that got them to this point are still not changed. By changing your habits and creating healthier and more nutritious habits, you can begin to see *real* change. In this book, I will discuss not only ways that you can use essential oils to create that change but also ways to use essential oils to block the munchies, curve the appetite, and help reduce the fat within your body.

Answer these questions prior to starting:

Have you been trying to lose weight, but your body is just not having it?

Have you ever considered essential oils as a method to help with your weight loss journey?

When considering healthier lifestyle changes, do you start to stress out and get overly anxious?

If you have thought about any of these questions at least once, then essential oils are the exact thing you will need to help you along your path to a healthy weight loss journey.

Although essential oils can only help with a small part of the weight loss journey, it is an especially useful part. Each essential oil that can be used for weight loss has a practical as well as medicinal benefit. Below, I will detail each oil and the benefit that it provides.

Grapefruit Oil

Metabolism is increased.

Rosemary Oil

Helps decrease your cortisol which lowers the stress levels that are associated with weight gain.

Fennel Oil

Energy levels are increased.

Orange Oil

Curbs your appetite and reduce the overeating that would put on the pounds.

Cinnamon Oil

Controls the blood sugar levels by aiding with the processing.

Sandalwood Oil

Suppresses negative and promote calm.

Bergamot Oil

The mind is clearer, and you are more awake.

Lavender Oil

Stress is calmed and anxiety is reduced.

Ginger Oil

Digestive Health aid.

Eucalyptus Oil

Stress and anxiety are alleviated.

Peppermint Oil

Appetite is suppressed.

Frankincense Oil

Speeds up your digestion with the production of bile and gastric juices.

Lemon Oil

Dissolves fat easily.

Jasmine Oil

Anxiety is reduced, the sex drive is increased, and depression and insomnia are reduced.

Now that you have learned which oils are best suited for weight loss, it is time to move on to some easy-to-follow recipes that will give you a better understanding of how to utilize them in your lifestyle. Weight loss is not easy, and it will not happen overnight. However, it will be much easier when you use essential oils to bring the results that you want without stressing about the outcome.

The next chapter walks you through several recipes for your home use. There is everything from:

- Weight loss recipes that are topical;
- Weight loss recipes that can be ingested;
- Weight loss recipes that are inhalants;
- **And so much more.**

With this, take out a notebook and a pen and start making notes about all the oils that are included in the next chapter and begin to incorporate the right recipes into your daily life and see an increase in the reduction of your weight.

You may not be happy right now with how much weight you have on you, but after a continuous use of this book and proper diet and exercise, you should see a drastic change begin to take shape!

Chapter 7: Easy-To-Follow Recipes for Weight Loss

Grapefruit Weight Loss Essential Oil Recipe

Add 2 drops of Grapefruit oil into your water and drink every day for a boost in your weight loss efforts. This should be done first thing in the morning. This boosts your metabolism as well as detoxifies your body and increases your loss in fat. This will help with the maintaining of weight loss. By drinking this concoction, you can relieve the bloating found in your stomach and digest your food easier.

Use an inhaler to get a direct result that that cravings when you are dieting. Grapefruit oil has a fresh and aromatic scent which can be harnessed by adding a few drops to an inhaler container or a cotton ball. Then, place it under your nose and breathe deeply. This helps with the parasympathetic nerve within the gastric region. This mechanism allows for the ghrelin to be activated for feeding induction. This is the process by which our body has cravings.

Topical application is a great way to utilize essential oils. You can apply them to the temples, wrists, chest, stomach, under the nose, and several other locations that would be benefited by this application. By using this application, you can curve the cravings as well as the appetite.

By adding a few drops of essential oil to a diffuser, you will be able to fight the cravings that are hitting you hard during those weight loss days and nights. These can be difficult times to get through—and fighting cravings is a must.

Using it in conjunction with a cellulite cream can help in fighting more of the inflammatory effects and uses bromelain to break that cellulite down much faster.

Cellulite Cream That Is All-Natural Using Grapefruit Essential Oil

Coconut oil-carrier oil (0.50c.)
Grapefruit Essential oil (15)
Glass jar for storage

Properly blend the Grapefruit with the coconut and store it in the storage jar that is glass. Use this rub to massage your areas with cellulite. You should massage for 5 minutes at a time. This will firm and reduce the cellulite.

Cinnamon Weight Loss Essential Oil Recipe

Place 2 drops into a glass water bottle or a cup of tea or coffee. You can also place 2 drops in tea, and some warm honey to help with the elimination of cravings and slow your appetite down. Add cinnamon to your baked goods as well so that you can incorporate these benefits into all your foods.

Use an inhaler and directly inhale a few drops of cinnamon into your olfactory senses. This will prevent you from having trouble with overeating, as well eliminate the cravings that you will definitely have at stressful times and at night. It will also help you to feel fuller inside and your mood will improve. If you are an emotional eater, then you will definitely benefit from this type of application.

Apply cinnamon as a topical application with a carrier oil and see the benefits of using this wonderful essential oil. Then use of jojoba, tamanu, or coconut oil is required since this is a topical application. You can run the application on your chest or your wrist.

Place a few drops into the diffuser and see how well your house smells afterward. You may also notice that you are not dealing with those midnight monster snack cravings. This will help your mood rise, and you will no longer feel snack-y or hungry due to emotions.

Ginger Weight Loss Essential Oil Recipe

Place a few drops of ginger essential oil into a glass of warm water and squeeze a few drops of lemon in with some honey that is raw. This will help with your weight loss journey and it tastes great.

Using an inhaler apply a few drops of Ginger inside the inhaler or on a cotton ball and use it to inhale when you are having cravings. This will also help you to slow down while eating and take your time. When you rush while you eat, you tend to eat more than is necessary since your stomach does not have time to catch up. This inhaler is also a great way to pick up your spirits.

Peppermint Weight Loss Essential Oil Recipe

Use a few drops of Peppermint oil in some water and drink this prior to eating a meal. This will help your appetite be suppressed. It is recommended to use a therapeutic brand of essential oil for any application that involved ingestion.

Inhaling a bit of Peppermint oil will not only remind you of Christmas time but also help to block your appetite when you are eating due to stress or emotions. This will also trigger your stomach to stop you from eating by triggering your full meter. Try this prior to eating to get the full benefit of this use.

Diffusing Peppermint oil in your home will make your house smell wonderful, and it will help you to not feel the need to eat. It is uplifting and blocks those cravings easily. It also provides you with the energy that is needed to be active throughout the day. This will motivate you to take on exercise or more activities. Which helps you to ultimately lose the weight.

Lemon Weight Loss Essential Oil Recipe

Add lemon to your water daily to help break down the fat and lose weight. This will help your digestive tract work properly and also aid in detoxifying your body from all the toxic chemicals that you have taken in while you ate unhealthy food choices.

Inhaling lemon is a great way to get a fresh, cooling scent and also block cravings that are sure to affect you. The great thing about lemons is that they will suppress your need to overeat, making you lose weight quickly.

Massages are a wonderful way to de-stress and add tension relief to your body. By using Lemon essential oil along with a carrier oil, you can get extra benefits. Massage this oil into the cellulite areas to reduce the cellulite, as well as eliminate the fat cells.

Inhaler Recipe for Weight Loss

Basil essential oil (3)

Lemon essential oil (4)

Oregano essential oil (3)

#2 Capsules for Weight Loss

Capsules Gelatin-Empty

Grapefruit essential oil (1)

Lemon essential oil (1)

Peppermint essential oil (1)

Olive oil (fill the space)

Making your capsules:

1. Using your oils place (1) per essential oil into each capsule.

2. Fill the remaining space with the olive oil.

3. Close your capsule and enjoy losing weight.

By taking one pill every day in the morning, you can begin to see changes in your eating habits and your weight will start to melt away. Then take another in the afternoon prior to eating lunch and you will increase your chances of losing weight exponentially.

Bergamot Weight Loss Essential Oil Recipe

Bergamot is a great oil to use within an inhaler. It provides a musty woody scent that helps to reduce the amount that you are eating by suppressing your need to eat more. This helps you lose weight and also gives you that wonderful aroma to smell.

By placing a few drops in your shower, you can get all the benefits of essential oils without the hassle of having to learn how to blend them. Make sure you plug your drain, so you do not lose your oil drops while showering. Inhale deeply for the benefits that are medicinal in nature as well as refreshing to the senses. This will get you to amplify your weight loss journey.

Diffuser Recipe for Weight Loss

Bergamot essential oil (3)
Geranium essential oil (3)
Mandarin essential oil (3)

Place this recipe into a diffuser to send that weight loss benefit all through your home or use it on a cotton ball or handkerchief as an inhaler that is personal to you. No one will know that you are working on losing weight until they start to see those pounds melt away. This will also help you get the sleep that is needed for a proper healthy lifestyle.

Sandalwood Weight Loss Essential Oil Recipe

Sandalwood is a wonderful oil to use in a diffuser or inhaler. You can place it on a cotton ball and inhale it under your nose or place a few drops in the diffuser and let the whole house benefit from it. This can stimulate a sense of relaxation and divert your mind to focus on something besides food. When you diffuse the oil, you will find that is a relaxing finish to a super long day.

Topical application can be done when working with Sandalwood, however, you will need a carrier oil when applying it. Anytime you feel like snacking on junk simply use your blended oil to cut those cravings by rubbing it on your wrists. You can also rub this on your ankles for a stressful day relief.

Lavender Weight Loss Essential Oil Recipe

Inhaling Lavender is calming and soothes the beast that lives within that craves junk. By using 2 or 3 drops you can focus on relieving those emotions that are causing you to be stressed or crave junk food. It provides a relaxing stress relief that decreases anxiety.

Diffusion of essential oils is one of the best ways to incorporate essential oils into your home. It brings a sense of peace and calm to the home and helps the inhabitants relax. By adding some drops of Lavender Oil, you will have an aroma that will travel throughout the whole house reducing temptations over food and anxious feelings around eating.

Inhaler for Weight Loss

Cotton ball or wicks
Inhaler cartridge
Lavender essential oil (15)

How to Prepare This Inhaler:

1. Using a glass dram place the lavender drops into the bowl and soak the cotton wicks or cotton balls in the bowl. Once they are thoroughly soaked place them in

the inhaler cartridge and utilize it to inhale that Lavender goodness that helps you lose weight.

Fennel Weight Loss Essential Oil Recipe

Fennel has a strong smell and can be added to a glass of water for the prevention of overeating. It can also aid you in digesting your food properly.

Another great way to use Fennel is to apply it topically with a carrier oil. Just a small dab on your wrist will block the craving to eat sugary things.

Inhaler for Weight Loss

Coconut oil-fractionated (1-oz.)
Fennel essential oil (18)
3% dilution

Preparing This Inhaler Recipe:

1. Mix your Fennel with the coconut oil and store it in a small glass bottle. This will provide a way for you to carry it around with you for easy access.

Eucalyptus Weight Loss Essential Oil Recipe

Inhaling Eucalyptus will help you feel much calmer and eliminate the need for that emotional eating that so many people do. When you emotionally eat it is due to stress, anxiety, fear, depression, or complacency. This will block the need to and also provide you with a great smelling home.

Eucalyptus has been known to help people breath better, but it also helps people feel refreshed and ready to take on the day. This creates a can-do attitude toward exercise, weight loss, and any other thing that you struggle facing day to day. Place a few drops in the bottom of your shower to start your day right.

Frankincense Weight Loss Essential Oil Recipe

Frankincense was one of the oils that was given to Baby Jesus and that has to say something about the value of its benefits, right. So, as you can guess, applying it to an inhaler and using it to lose weight is not a far stretch. Frankincense has been known to create an atmosphere of calm and help relax the mind so that you do not emotionally eat.

Applying a few drops into a diffuser will help to let your whole home smell of earth nature. It creates a refreshing scent and also induces the feeling that calms your nervous system down. This blocks you from eating unnecessary snacks and leads to stress relief and anxiety reduction after long hard days. This increases the reduction of cravings.

Jasmine Weight Loss Essential Oil Recipe

Jasmine oil is a wonderful and floral aroma that is great for inhalers since it prevents the act of overeating. Place a few drops on some tissue or handkerchief to keep on you all day long. If you feel anxious you can use this to calm your feelings and reduce your stress.

A diffuser is another great way to help with your weight loss journey. By adding jasmine (3) and grapefruit (5) to your diffuser you will have a citrus aroma that is refreshing and calming. It also provides a relaxing way to relax the parasympathetic nerve that is housed in the gastric system. This will prevent you from dealing with cravings which makes it a great way to lose weight.

Orange Weight Loss Essential Oil Recipe

Orange is a great citrus scent that many people enjoy smelling. It provides you with some perking up since it energizes your senses as well as stimulating your senses with the pleasing aroma and reducing your need to overeat. By inhaling it you can have a go-to remedy while out that is pleasing to the nose.

Placing a few drops of Orange oil in some water and drinking this during meals will help to curb your intake of food. This provides a way for your stomach to intuitively know when you are full and block you from eating too much. Orange oil is great as a weight loss supplement.

Rosemary Weight Loss Essential Oil Recipe

Rosemary is a great addition to any meal, especially Italian system meals. What many people do not know is that it is also great for reducing the levels of cortisol within your body which is what makes you feel stress. The psychology behind this is when you are less stressed out you will eat less food. So, by being less stressed you can begin to reduce your intake of food and lose weight. This will trim your waistline in no time.

More Recipes to Help You with Your Weight Loss Efforts

Additional Recipe # 1

What is needed:

Home diffuser

Lavender essential oil (5)

Vetiver essential oil (4)

Place a few drops within the diffuser and turn the diffuser on prior to going to bed. This should run for 15 minutes and then have 1 hour of off time. This is a powerful anti-inflammatory that helps with the reduction of inflammation in the joints. This will help you with chronic inflammation as well as weight loss.

Additional Recipe # 2

What is needed:

Diffuser for your home

Roman chamomile essential oil

Diffusing the Roman Chamomile oil in your diffuser will add anti-inflammatory properties to your weight loss journey. The less inflamed your body is the less you will eat.

Few Key Recipes That Can Help with Your Weight Loss Journey

Peppermint

Peppermint is a pain relief and stomach ache reliever. It also provides a cool effect that will help with fevers. By rubbing your temples, you can see drastic improvements. When you diffuse peppermint oil in your home you will feel energy quickly as well as a boost in your activity level.

Add 10 drops to the bath and soak in the water for a relief form achy muscles. Add 2 to a glass of water for a minty fresh breath experience and include some in your toothpaste for a refreshing flavor in your mouth.

Lemon

Lemon is great for salads as well as smoothies, so adding 3 drops to your water is also a great idea. Diffuse it in your home for a clean aroma or at work for an energizing experience. If you experience some grogginess during the day you should try inhaling some lemon to get a pick me up throughout the day.

Grapefruit

Adding 3 drops to a glass of water is a great way to lose weight. You can also massage your body with some grapefruit oil and experience a refreshing aroma as you are getting some much-needed relief. Diffuse this oil in your home for a cleaner and fresher air as well as a way to block those cravings.

Ginger

Add a few drops of this oil to your tea or a smoothie that is green. This is a great way to get the added benefits of the ginger into your day. You can also diffuse the oil in your home and experience a spicy aroma that will help alleviate any stomach problems.

Citrus Mix

- mood elevating

- uplifting

- Fat burning

- energizing

What You Will Need:
Lemon essential oil (3)
Lime essential oil (3)
Bergamot essential oil (3)
Coconut oil (0.50c.)

Preparing the recipe:
1. Combine your essential oils into a glass dram and twirl the oils to blend them. Then pour in the coconut oil and twirl it again.

2. Next, use your oil for massages by adding to a lotion, or perfumes by adding to a spray bottle.

Peppermint/Lavender Blend for Calming

- Calming

- Anxiety reducing

- Relaxing

- Appetite curbing

What You Will Need:

Coconut oil (0.50c.)

Lavender essential oil (5)

Rosemary essential oil (5)

Preparing This Essential Oil Blend:

1. Blend the oils together in a glass dram and then add in the coconut oil, twirling to blend the oils together.

2. Once blended add to the sternum for blocking the junk food cravings that you will experience while dieting. You can also use this to relieve anxiety.

Invigorating Sandalwood/Cinnamon Diffuser Oil Recipe

- Warming
- Uplifting
- Energizing

What You Will Need:

Water-purified (0.25c.)

Sandalwood essential oil (4)

Cinnamon essential oil (2)

Preparing This Essential Oil Blend:

1. Blend the oils together in a glass dram, twirling to blend the oils together.

2. Once blended add the oils to a diffuser with the purified water and turn it on for 15 minutes, then off for at least an hour.

3. This creates a warming effect that motivates you to hit the gym or be more active.

Lemon Elixir

- Detoxification

- Digestive Aid

What You Will Need:
Water-purified (12 -oz.)
Lemon essential oil (5)

Preparing This Essential Oil Blend:
1. Add the lemon drops to the 12 oz. of water and drink first thing in the morning.

2. Lemon will help with detoxifying your body. This helps to increase the activity in your life and also aids with digestion. Drink this daily for optimal health and weight loss.

Grapefruit Topical Energizing Balm

- Boosts moods

- Appetite curbing

What You Will Need:

Carrier oil (0.50c.)

Grapefruit essential oil (5)

Preparing This Essential Oil Blend:

1. Blend the oil with the carrier oil and store in a glass container.

2. Use this balm to help with your weight loss needs.

3. This balm stores at room temperature for 6 months or less.

Peppermint Shower

- Calming
- Anxiety reducing
- Relaxing
- Appetite curbing

What You Will Need:

Peppermint essential oil (5)

Preparing This Essential Oil Blend:

1. Drop a few drops of peppermint in the shower the next time you are in there. This will promote weight loss as well as sooth your stomach when feeling sick. The minty scent will be intoxicating as well.

Ginger Lemonade for Digestion

- Calming

- Anxiety reducing

- Relaxing

- Appetite curbing

What You Will Need:
Water (12-oz.)
Honey (1tsp)
Lemon essential oil (1)
Ginger essential oil (1)

Preparing This Essential Oil Blend:
1. Blend the lemon with the ginger in a cold glass of water every morning.

2. Use the honey to sweeten it for your favorite flavor and a delicious ginger lemonade for digestion.

3. Enjoy one per day for delicious goodness and weight loss benefits.

Cinnamon Infusion for the Stove Top

- Craving elimination
- Warming
- Inviting
- Holiday festive

What You Will Need:

Water (6c)

Cinnamon essential oil (10)

Preparing This Essential Oil Blend:

1. Place your water in your pot and turn the stove on.
2. Drop in the cinnamon oil and let it boil for 2 hours.
3. Let it sit and as it cools it will infuse the whole house with that cinnamon goodness.
4. This is excellent for winter time and holiday seasons.

Lavender Mist

- Calming
- Anxiety reducing
- Stress relief
- Appetite curbing

What You Will Need:
Water (12-oz.)
Spray bottle-glass
Lavender essential oil (15)

Preparing This Essential Oil Blend:
1. Apply water to the spray bottle and add in the lavender oil. Then use it to spray the rooms with the aroma of lavender.

Green Tea That is Uplifting

- Appetite curbing

- Digestion Aid

What You Will Need:
Water (2c.)
Honey (1tsp)
Ginger essential oil (1)

Preparing This Essential Oil Blend:

1. Boil the cups of water prior to adding the drops.

2. Add the drops to the water and then the honey for sweetening it.

3. Drink a cup prior to eating a meal as well as right after eating a meal. You should also drink one when eating snacks as well. this will provide proper digestion.

Fennel Quencher

- Quenches your thirst
- Health benefits
- Curves cravings
- Appetite curbing

What You Will Need:
Water (1gal)
Honey (1tsp)
Fennel essential oil (2)

Preparing This Essential Oil Blend:
1. After exercise place 2 drops of fennel in a 1-gallon pitcher of water and drink up.
2. The use of fennel will not be overpowering since it is a large amount of water with a small amount of fennel.

Cardamom Elixir Prior to Dinner

- Digestive support

What You Will Need:

Water (12-oz.)

Honey (1tsp)

Cardamom essential oil (3)

Preparing This Essential Oil Blend:

1. After exercise place 2 drops of Cardamom in a 1-gallon pitcher of water and drink up.

2. The use of Cardamom will not be overpowering since it is a large amount of water with a small amount of Cardamom.

Citrus Massage Balm and Oil

- Energy Boost

- Weight loss benefits

- Burns fat

What You Will Need:

Carrier oil (1c.)

Orange essential oil (5)

Lemon essential oil (5)

Grapefruit essential oil (5)

Preparing This Essential Oil Blend:

1. Blend your oils together and twirl them for proper blending.

2. Then, add them to the carrier oil of your choice.

3. Next, store this recipe in a container that is glass and can be used later.

4. Rub this balm on the parts that bother you the most.

Weight Loss Pills Natural Remedies # 1

- Digestive support

What You Will Need:

Coconut Oil-Fractionated (12)

Lemon essential oil (2)

Grapefruit essential oil (2)

Peppermint essential oil (2)

Empty Capsule-vegetable

Preparing This Essential Oil Blend:

1. Blend the essential oils in a glass dram, then twirl it to ensure proper blending.

2. Pour the coconut oil in to the mix and twirl it to blend properly.

3. Once blended fill your vegetable capsule.

4. Take a pill per day for breakfast to increase weight loss.

5. Prepare a week worth in advance for easier application.

Weight Loss Pills Natural Remedy # 2

- Digestive support

What You Will Need:

Coconut Oil-Fractionated (12)

Cinnamon essential oil (2)

Lemon essential oil (2)

Black pepper essential oil (2)

Grapefruit essential oil (2)

Peppermint essential oil (2)

Empty Capsule-vegetable

Preparing This Essential Oil Blend:

1. Blend the essential oils in a glass dram, then twirl it to ensure proper blending.

2. Pour the coconut oil in to the mix and twirl it to blend properly.

3. Once blended fill your vegetable capsule.

4. Take a pill per day for breakfast to increase weight loss.

5. Prepare a week worth in advance for easier application.

Diffuser Blend for Curbing Appetite # 1

- Curb appetite

- Cravings reduced

- Reduces overeating

What You Will Need:

Water (4oz)

Lemon essential oil (3)

Ylang-Ylang essential oil (1)

Grapefruit essential oil (3)

Spearmint essential oil (1)

Preparing This Essential Oil Blend:

1. Blend the essential oils in a glass dram, then twirl it to ensure proper blending.

2. Pour them into the diffuser with the 4 oz. of water.

3. Turn on the diffuser and diffuse for 15 minutes, then let it sit for 1 hour.

Diffuser Blend for Curbing Appetite # 2

- Curb appetite
- Cravings reduced
- Reduces overeating

What You Will Need:

Water (4oz)

Lemon essential oil (3)

Rose essential oil (1)

Grapefruit essential oil (3)

Spearmint essential oil (1)

Preparing This Essential Oil Blend:

1. Blend the essential oils in a glass dram, then twirl it to ensure proper blending.

2. Pour them into the diffuser with the 4 oz. of water.

3. Turn on the diffuser and diffuse for 15 minutes, then let it sit for 1 hour.

Water Infusion

- Curb appetite

- Cravings reduced

- Reduces overeating

What You Will Need:

Water (4oz)

Grapefruit essential oil (8)

Preparing This Essential Oil Blend:

1. Pour the grapefruit oil into the 2 liters of water for drinking prior to every meal.

2. This will increase your weight loss efforts.

Weight Loss Foot Rub

- Curb appetite
- Cravings reduced
- Reduces overeating

What You Will Need:

Carrier oil (2tsp)

Lavender essential oil (4)

Juniper essential oil (3)

Cypress essential oil (5)

Grapefruit essential oil (8)

Basil essential oil (4)

Preparing This Essential Oil Blend:

1. Add all of the oils into a dram and twirl to blend them.
2. Next, blend them with the carrier oil.
3. Once they are blended place in your glass bottle for storage.
4. Use as a foot rub prior to bedtime or add to the bath for a weight loss boost.

Massage Oil for Weight loss

- Curb appetite

- Cravings reduced

- Reduces overeating

What You Will Need:

Carrier oil (1-oz)

Grapefruit essential oil (40)

Geranium essential oil (30)

Rose essential oil (30)

Lemon essential oil (30)

Preparing This Essential Oil Blend:

1. Blend all the oils together in a glass dram.

2. Twirl them to ensure proper blending.

3. Then, add in the carrier oil.

4. Twirl the ingredients to blend fully.

5. Massage on your skin after a hot bath or use for a professional session at a massage studio. This will increase your weight loss efforts.

Anti-Cellulite Rub

- Curb appetite

- Cravings reduced

- Reduces overeating

What You Will Need:

Coconut oil (0.75c)

Lemon essential oil (10)

Witch Hazel (2tbsp)

Beeswax (2tbsp)

Grapefruit essential oil (30)

Basil essential oil (4)

Preparing This Essential Oil Blend:

1. Blend your witch hazel with the essential oils in a glass bowl that is small.

2. Melt the coconut oil with the beeswax and blend it with the witch hazel.

3. Stir them gently to blend properly.

4. Move the mix to a glass jar that is small.

5. Store in a cool and dry location for optimal use.

6. Let it sit for 3 hours before using.

7. Use this on your cellulite every day in order to reduce the skins puckered effect. This will be a great help after weight loss.

Tummy Tuck No More Rub

- Improve the texture of the skin
- Help with weight loss

What You Will Need:

EVOO (1c)

Lavender essential oil (15)

Frankincense essential oil (15)

Geranium (15)

Rosewater (1c)

Grapefruit essential oil (15)

Beeswax (0.25c)

Vitamin E (0.333c)

Preparing This Essential Oil Blend:

1. Place the ingredients minus the rose water and essential oils in a boiler that is doubled.
2. Warm up the mix and melt them over medium heat.
3. Pour this blend into a processor letting it cool prior to blending.
4. Blend slowly while you add the rose water, emulsifying the blend.

5. Add in the essential oil one by one and then quickly blend it all together. This creates the mix.

6. Pour this mix into a container that is sealable and made of glass.

7. Use to rub the abdomen for tighter skin. This will also help reduce the fat as well as any bloating that you have.

Massage Blends for Weight Loss

Reduce the Fat

Grapefruit essential oil (5)

Almond oil (0.25c)

Lemon essential oil (5)

Cypress essential oil (5)

Preparation method:

Mix together all the oils and blend properly.

Anti-Cellulite Rub

Grapefruit essential oil (10)

Cypress essential oil (2)

Ginger essential oil (2)

Rosemary essential oil (5)

Peppermint essential oil (2)

Carrier oil (2 tsp)

Preparation method:

1. Blend all the essential oils together in a glass dram, then twirl it to blend.

2. Add in the carrier oil and blend together.

3. Store in a container for later use.

4. Apply to your body when you need it.

Rejuvenation Bath

Grapefruit essential oil (5)

Lemon essential oil (5)

Ginger essential oil (5)

Sandalwood essential oil (5)

Orange essential oil (5)

Preparation Method:

1. Run a hot bath.

2. Pour the oils together and the twirl it to blend properly.

3. Once the bath is ready, pour in your oils, and then swirl the bath water.

4. Soak in the tub for 15 minutes.

Suppress the Appetite Diffuser

Grapefruit essential oil (5)

Mandarin essential oil (40)

Ginger essential oil (12)

Lemon essential oil (20)

Peppermint essential oil (12)

Preparation Method:

1. Blend the oils together by pouring them into a glass dram and twirling the dram.

2. Pour 4-fl. oz. of water into the diffuser.

3. Pour in the essential oils.

4. Turn it on for 15 minutes at a time.

Rejuvenation Bath

Grapefruit essential oil (5)

Lemon essential oil (5)

Ginger essential oil (5)

Sandalwood essential oil (5)

Orange essential oil (5)

Preparation Method:

1. Run a hot bath.

2. Pour the oils together and the twirl it to blend properly.

3. Once the bath is ready, pour in your oils, and then swirl the bath water.

4. Soak in the tub for 15 minutes.

Other Massage Blends

Diffusion Appetite-Suppressing

(8) bergamot essential oil

(2) ginger essential oil

(5) grapefruit essential oil

Massage to Fighting Fat # 1

(5) grapefruit essential oil

(5) cypress essential oil

(5) lemon essential oil

Massage for Fighting Fat # 2

(5) ginger essential oil

(5) rosemary essential oil

(2) peppermint essential oil

(3) cinnamon essential oil

Massage for Cellulite Busting

(7) grapefruit essential oil

(3) juniper essential oil

(5) cypress essential oil

Now that I have given you a basis of recipes to get you started it is time to collect the oils that you will need and to examine the precautions that could take place if they are not properly applied.

What you can expect from the next chapter is the safety precautions that are important to your safety and the safety of others around you. If you are not sure about something do some research or check into more information with a licensed aromatherapist. They should be able to help you locate the appropriate weight loss recipe that will fit your needs.

Chapter 8: Safety Measures and Precautions to Take When Using Essential Oils for Weight Loss

Essential oils should be safely stored and out of the reach of children. If the oils are exposed to light during storage, they will deteriorate fast. Use a cool, dark storage environment. Refrigerating the oils will decrease the rate at which they spoil. Tightly close all bottles. This will prevent the evaporation of the oils as well as oxidization. Oils can ruin the furniture—be careful when handling them.

The essential oils that are refined have a lifespan of one-year, while unrefined essential oils' lifespan would be much shorter. Storing the unrefined ones in the fridge extends their lifespan a bit. Most oils will be fine for 1 to 2 years if safely stored—citrus will only be fine for 6 to 9 months due to storage and usage.

Medication for an ailment is located in every single person's medicine cabinet, so why not essential oils? Prior to using essential oils, make sure that the oils you are using will not interact with your conditions or medications. This means that patients with low blood pressure as well as patients with heart conditions do not need to use grapefruit oil. Pregnant and nursing moms as well as their babies should never use Tea tree oil.

Testing for Allergies

To test to make sure that you are not allergic to any of the oils that you will be using, use these steps:

- Rub the carrier oil on your chest

- Sit for 12 hours with it on there and wait.

- Look for itchy, red patchy, irritated skin.

If you see no irritation, proceed to testing the essential oils on top of the carrier oil.

- Add 1 drop of the chosen essential oil with the 15 drops of non-allergic carrier oil.

- When you receive no reaction, you are fine and can continue to use that oil.

Oils should never be applied to any of the locations below. If you do get them in those areas, take immediate action.

- The lips

- The eyes

- Sensitive parts

- The genitals

To flush oil out of your eyes, use water or sweet almond oil—applied directly on the eyes. This will neutralize the oil.

Drinking alcohol is not recommended when using essential oils in your life, but you do not have to miss that dinner time wine glass.

Sunlight can be quite painful if exposed too soon after using a citrus oil, so avoid it for 30 minutes.

When you use these oils on your skin, be extra careful and take precautions. They can be irritating, so use them sparingly:

- Lemon
- Spearmint
- Black Pepper
- Clove
- Melissa
- Grapefruit
- Mandarin

- Lemongrass
- Orange
- Cinnamon
- Peppermint

If you have super sensitive skin, then the most optimal application method would be to apply them only to your bath. This will dilute the oils and prevent you from being affected negatively by the oils.

You would apply the oil to these locations for headache relief:

- Temples
- Behind the ears
- Forehead

You would apply the oils for relieving a stomach problem to these locations:

- The stomach
- The abdomen

You would apply the oils to relieve a fever to these locations:

- The forehead
- On the temples

- Behind the neck
- Under the feet
- Behind the ears

You would apply the oil to relieve sore muscles to these locations:
- Apply oil to the muscles that are most bothering you.

You would apply the oil to relieve sleeping problems to these locations:
- Under the feet
- Behind your ears
- neck

You would apply the oils to help someone, throughout the day, feel calmer to these locations:
- The temples
- The wrist
- Behind your ears

You would apply the oils to relieve a chest congestion or a cough to these locations:
- chest

- under the nose
- diffuser

you would apply the oil for flue or influenza to these locations:

- spine
- lungs area
- back of the neck
- diffuser
- under the nose

The next chapter will be all about properly applying the essential oils based on your weight loss journey. I know that many of you are worried about whether or not essential oils can help you in this particular aspect. The simple answer to this is that with time and patience, you will begin to see the benefits that weight loss using essential oils has for you. Consider the application methods and how they will affect you. Then, consider the oils that you will be using, and finally decide which ones are the most accommodating for your lifestyle.

Then, move forward with your weight loss journey by utilizing all the tools that have been provided for you within this book as well as all the tools that are provided for you through a traditional weight loss method.

Do not forget that outside of actual exercise, both proper dieting and a healthy mindset are a must—there is no alternative to hard work.

Chapter 9: Properly Applying Essential Oils in Your Weight Loss Routine

With all methods of using essential oils, you will need to know the proper way to apply them.

To apply oils for a regular application, you will need to apply them around these locations:

- Ears
- Temples
- Back of neck
- Wrists
- Forehead
- Under the feet

For any other application that is specific, you will need to apply in the location that is most affecting you.

If the oils are being applied topically, you will need to blend them with a carrier oil. Carrier oils that can be used are:

- Jojoba

- Coconut
- Almond
- Witch hazel
- Olive oil
- Grapeseed
- Aloe Vera
- And any other oil that is ok for essential oil blending.

Other application methods include:
- Baths
- Inhalers
- Diffusers
- Ingestion (food grade)
- Aromatic lamps

After you have applied your oils, you need to follow up on your application site to make sure you have no adverse reaction.

Weight loss programs can utilize many of the essential oils that are on the market. If you are fully ready to lose that weight, then consider incorporating essential oils into your weight loss regime.

Remember that essential oils all have properties that can interfere with the sensitive skins that are located on our bodies. If you apply something to your skin and it is itchy, irritated, or red—you should immediately apply almond oil or water.

I have spent numerous hours compiling the details in this and providing a way for those that wish to use essential oils for weight loss the ability to use them in a proper way. Essential oils are a great investment to make. Not only do they provide benefits for weight loss, but they also provide an amazing way for you to maintain your family's health and well-being. The great thing about the weight loss essential oils is that children who are suffering from being overweight are capable of utilizing about every single oil within these recipes. This provides a whole family of weight loss regimen that allows for each person to utilize the benefits of essential oils to get healthy and *stay* healthy.

What else in the world could beat the benefits that essential oils can provide for not only you but also your children, your pets, and your home?

I believe that essential oils will be utilized for years to come due to the magnificent benefits they provide. Now, get out there and start losing weight in a healthy way!

Chapter 10: Easy-to-Follow Recipes that can help with Health Issues

Below I will go over several easy to follow recipes for Kids, women, and Men that can be used to alleviate any ailment that you may be faced with. Each recipe will have a dilution ratio, as well as a proper mixing instruction and the specific use that it can be used for. There will be several blends that will need to be blended properly for optimal results.

For Kids

When creating a blend for children you want to dilute your oils by a 0.5 to 1% solution, with 3-6 drops per ounce of your favorite carrier oil. This is ideal for those under the age of 5. For kids over the age of five a 2% dilution is safe. Check with the Primary care provider for a contraindication of medications already being taken.

There are several recipes that can be used in a roller ball type application, and these can be used for everyday use. However, there are a few that are good for having on hand for the occasional need. It is recommended to not use specific mentholated oils on children that are young or have trouble breathing when around mentholated products.

Sleep Issues

Supplies that you will need:

Lavender Essential Oils

Vetiver Essential Oils

Roman chamomile Essential Oil

Your 10-15 mL roller ball applicator

Your favorite carrier oils

Glass dram for blending with a pour spout

Directions for blending:
1. In order to prepare this blend properly, you will need to have a glass dram to use for preparation prior to placing it in the roller bottle. Using the oils start with the lavender oil and drop 3 drops into the dram.
2. The use the Vetiver and drop in 2 drops
3. Next, add in the Roman chamomile at 2 drops.
4. Roll the dram in the palms of your hands to blend the oils together.
5. Then, pour into your roller ball applicator.
6. Once you have poured in your blended Essential oils, use your carrier oil and fill the remaining space with the oil.
7. Place the lid on the roller ball and roll the ball between your hands a couple of times, then rotate the

bottle using your first finger and thumb in an up and down motion.
8. This will help the oils to blend properly.

To apply:

Apply to the bottom of your children; feet in the arch, behind their ears, and across the back of their neck. This will help them to sleep. *It is best to start with one application location and then move on to more locations as the oil concentrate is not fully helpful with just the one.

Easier Breathing

Supplies that you will need:

Rosemary Essential Oils

Cardamom Essential Oil

Peppermint Essential Oil

Eucalyptus Essential Oils

Lemon Essential Oil

Tea Tree Essential Oil

Your 10-15 mL roller ball applicator

Your favorite carrier oils

Glass dram for blending with a pour spout

Directions for blending:
1. In order to prepare this blend properly, you will need to have a glass dram to use for preparation prior to placing it in the roller bottle. Using the oils start with the Peppermint oil and drop 2 drops into the dram.
2. The use the Cardamom and drop in 1 drop.
3. Next, add in the Tea Tree, Lemon, Rosemary, and Eucalyptus oils at 1 drop each.
4. Roll the dram in the palms of your hands to blend the oils together.
5. Then, pour into your roller ball applicator.

6. Once you have poured in your blended Essential oils, use your carrier oil and fill the remaining space with the oil.
7. Place the lid on the roller ball and roll the ball between your hands a couple of times, then rotate the bottle using your first finger and thumb in an up and down motion.
8. This will help the oils to blend properly.

To apply:

Apply to the bottom of your children's feet in the arch, as well as their chest to aid with the reduction of a cough or chest congestion. This will help them to have an easier time breathing. *It is best to start with one application location and then move on to more locations as the oil concentrate is not fully helpful with just the one.

Insect Bites Spray

Supplies that you will need:

Lemon Essential Oils

Juniper berries Essential Oil

Borage Essential Oil

Tea Tree Essential Oils

Glass spray bottle

Your favorite carrier oils

Glass dram for blending with a pour spout

Directions for blending:
1. In order to prepare this blend properly, you will need to have a glass dram to use for preparation prior to placing it in the spray bottle. Using the oils start with the Borage oil add 1 tsp to the dram.
2. Then, use the Tea Tree Oil and Juniper Berries Oil and drop in 2 drops each into the dram.
3. Next, add in the Lemon Oil at 1 drop each.
4. Roll the dram in the palms of your hands to blend the oils together.
5. Then, pour into your glass spray bottle.
6. Once you have poured in your blended Essential oils, use your carrier oil and fill the remaining space with the oil.

7. Place the lid on the spray lid on the bottle and roll the ball between your hands a couple of times, then rotate the bottle using your first finger and thumb in an up and down motion.
8. This will help the oils to blend properly.

To apply:

To apply this treatment, you would need to verify that your child is not allergic to any of the ingredients first. Then once you have verified their ability to use the oil spray, you should spray it on the insect bite as needed for itch and pain from stinging,

Lice Be-gone

Supplies that you will need:
Ginger Essential Oils
Walnut Essential Oil
Peppermint Essential Oil
Lavender Essential Oils
Your favorite carrier oils
Glass container that is sealable for storage
Glass dram for blending with a pour spout

Directions for blending:
1. In order to prepare this blend properly, you will need to have a glass dram to use for preparation prior to placing it in the sealable glass jar for later use. Using the oils start with the walnut oil and pour 1 tsp into the dram.
2. The use the Peppermint, Lavender, and Ginger dropping 5 drops each into the dram.
3. Roll the dram in the palms of your hands to blend the oils together.
4. Once you have blended the Essential oils, you are able to use this treatment to kill off lice and get them gone.
5. Place the oil into a glass sealable container and place that container between your hands and roll a couple

of times, then rotate the bottle using your first finger and thumb in an up down motion.
6. This will help the oils to blend properly.

To apply:

Ensure that your child is not allergic to any of these oils prior to use. Apply to the hair on your child's head, and massage it into the scalp. Then place the head in a night cap or shower cap and let them sleep with it on their head. Follow this procedure nightly until there is not more bugs and knits.

For Women

Women deal with lots of ailments throughout their day. They can have arthritis, PMS, anxiety, Depression, Endometriosis, and even headaches on a daily basis.

PMS Bath

Supplies that you will need:
Bergamot Essential Oils
Palmarosa Essential Oil
Geranium Essential Oil
Glass container with a sealable lid
Your favorite carrier oils
Glass dram for blending with a pour spout

Directions for blending:
1. In order to prepare this blend properly, you will need to have a glass dram to use for preparation prior to placing it in the roller bottle. Using the oils start with the Geranium, Bergamot, and Palmarosa oil and drop 5 drops of each into the dram.
2. Roll the dram in the palms of your hands to blend the oils together.
3. Then, pour into your storage container that is glass.

4. Once you have poured in your blended Essential oils, use your carrier oil and fill the remaining space with the oil.
5. Place the lid on the storage container and roll the container between your hands a couple of times, then rotate the bottle using your first finger and thumb in an up and down motion.
6. This will help the oils to blend properly.

To apply:
Ensure that you are not allergic to any of the ingredients found in this recipe. Prepare a bath and add a cap full of Epsom salt, once it is fully dissolved pour in the oils and use your hand to blend it through the water. Climb into the bath and soak for 30 minutes in the bath with the oils and Epsom salt.

Deodorant for Women

Supplies that you will need:

Lavender Essential Oils

Tolu Balsam

Jojoba oil

Cornstarch

Glass container with a sealable lid

Your favorite carrier oils

Glass dram for blending with a pour spout

Directions for blending:
1. In order to prepare this blend properly, you will need to have a glass dram to use for preparation prior to placing the storage container. Using the oils start with the Tolu Balsam oil and drop 3 drops of each into the dram.
2. The pour in 2 drops of Lavender oil.
3. Roll the dram in the palms of your hands to blend the oils together.
4. Then, pour into your storage container that is glass.

To apply:
Using the jojoba oil rub your underarms 30 minutes after you have shaved. Then rub the oil into the underarm area. Once this is fully rubbed in, use a towel to dry the excess oil.

Next, use the cornstarch to dab the oil with and dry it out fully. This should provide you 2 days of freshness and clean smelling underarms.

Hair Tonic for Women with Oily Hair

Supplies that you will need:

Grapeseed Oils

Lime Essential Oil

Rosemary Essential Oil

Ylang-Ylang Essential Oils

Glass spray bottle

Glass dram for blending with a pour spout

Directions for blending:
1. In order to prepare this blend properly, you will need to have a glass dram to use for preparation prior to placing it in the spray bottle. Using the oils start with the Ylang-Ylang, as well as Lime and drop 9 drops of each into the dram.
2. Then drop the rosemary into the dram using 8 drops.
3. Roll the dram in the palms of your hands to blend the oils together.
4. Then, pour into your glass spray bottle.
5. Once you have poured in your blended Essential oils, use your carrier oil and fill the remaining space with the oil.
6. Place the sprayer on the spray bottle and roll the container between your hands a couple of times, then

rotate the bottle using your first finger and thumb in an up and down motion.
7. This will help the oils to blend properly.

To apply:

Ensure that you are not allergic to any of the ingredients found in this recipe. Spray your head with the oil mixture using only about 1 tsp on your scalp. Massage into the scalp. Leaving it on overnight is best but several hours is ok as well. Place a towel or shower cap over your head allowing the oil to soak into your scalp and hair. Once you are ready to wash it off wash your hair twice to remove the oil with warm water. It is best to use organic shampoo at this time. Continue using this hair tonic until you have reached the hair goals that you have. Your hair needs to be full, shiny, and soft.

Reduce that Cellulite

Supplies that you will need:

Lemon Essential Oils

Fennel Essential Oil

Benzoin Essential Oil

Rosemary Essential Oil

Glass container with a sealable lid

Your favorite carrier oils

Glass dram for blending with a pour spout

Directions for blending:
1. In order to prepare this blend properly, you will need to have a glass dram to use for preparation prior to placing it in the storage container. Using the oils start with the blending of Fennel, Benzoin, rosemary, and Lemon with 5 drops each into the dram.
2. Roll the dram in the palms of your hands to blend the oils together.
3. Then, pour into your storage container that is glass.
4. Once you have poured in your blended Essential oils, use your carrier oil and place 4 tsp. into the container.
5. Place the lid on the storage container and roll the container between your hands a couple of times, then rotate the bottle using your first finger and thumb in an up and down motion.

6. This will help the oils to blend properly.

To apply:

Ensure that you are not allergic to any of the ingredients found in this recipe. When you are just getting out of the shower, massage this ointment on the areas that are covered with cellulite. This will help reduce the lines and dimples that are found in skin that has been stretch taught from excess weight. Add in a healthy diet and you will combat the cellulite on both levels.

For Men

Men deal with different but similar issues to women. They will have sore muscle related to hard manual labor done on a busy day, or a migraine headache due to the stress of pressure at work. They also experience PMS symptoms; however, it is in a much different way than how Women feel it. This doesn't mean that men are excluded from using the recipes above for women but there are a few other recipes that could be used for men that go right along with the ones for women.

Sore Muscles

Supplies that you will need:
Nutmeg Essential Oils
Ylang-Ylang Essential Oil
Ginger Essential Oil
Rosemary Essential Oil
Glass container with a sealable lid
Your favorite carrier oils
Glass dram for blending with a pour spout

Directions for blending:
1. In order to prepare this blend properly, you will need to have a glass dram to use for preparation prior to

placing it in the storage bottle. Using the Ginger and the Ylang-Ylang oils start by adding 5 drops of each into the dram.
2. Then, add in the Nutmeg with 3 drops into the dram.
3. Next, place 2 drops of Rosemary into the dram.
4. Roll the dram in the palms of your hands to blend the oils together.
5. Then, pour into your storage container that is glass.
6. Once you have poured in your blended Essential oils, use your carrier oil and pour 1 tablespoon into the container.
7. Place the lid on the storage container and roll the container between your hands a couple of times, then rotate the bottle using your first finger and thumb in an up and down motion.
8. This will help the oils to blend properly.

To apply:
Ensure that you are not allergic to any of the ingredients found in this recipe. When you are experiencing soreness in your muscles pull this storage container out and massage the oil blend onto the muscles that are aching. This will add an anti-inflammatory to your muscles and help relieve the soreness, the tightness, and the pressure.

Strength and Endurance Rub

Supplies that you will need:

Peppermint Essential Oils

Grapefruit Essential Oil

Ginger Essential Oil

Lemon Essential Oil

Thyme Essential Oil

Celery Essential Oil

Glass container with a sealable lid

Grapeseed oil

Glass dram for blending with a pour spout

Directions for blending:
1. In order to prepare this blend properly, you will need to have a glass dram to use for preparation prior to placing it in the glass storage bottle. Using the oils start with the ginger oil and drop 6 drops of each into the dram.
2. Then, apply 5 drops of the thyme, Celery, Peppermint, and Grapefruit oil into the dram.
3. Next, add in 4 drops of the lemon oil.
4. Roll the dram in the palms of your hands to blend the oils together.
5. Then, pour into your storage container that is glass.

6. Once you have poured in your blended Essential oils, use your Grapeseed oil and add in 2 tablespoons.
7. Place the lid on the storage container and roll the container between your hands a couple of times, then rotate the bottle using your first finger and thumb in an up and down motion.
8. This will help the oils to blend properly.

To apply:
Ensure that you are not allergic to any of the ingredients found in this recipe.

Complete an exercise to test the changes that will be taking place after using this ointment. Massage the blend into those muscles that you will be targeting. Wait for around 2 hours to repeat that same exercise and make a record of the results that you receive. By using the oil for 7 days in this same manner you should be able to see improvements over time that is noticeable.

Snoring be Gone

Supplies that you will need:
Lavender Essential Oils
Marjoram Essential Oil
Petitgrain Essential Oil
Cajaput Essential Oil
Chamomile Essential Oil
Myrtle Essential Oil
Glass container with a sealable lid
Your favorite carrier oils
Glass dram for blending with a pour spout

Directions for blending:
1. In order to prepare this blend properly, you will need to have a glass dram to use for preparation prior to placing it in the glass container. Using the oils start with the Myrtle and the Cajaput oil by dropping 4 drops of each into the dram.
2. Then, drop 3 drops of the Lavender, Chamomile, Petitgrain, and Marjoram into the dram.
3. Roll the dram in the palms of your hands to blend the oils together.
4. Then, pour into your storage container that is glass.

5. Once you have poured in your blended Essential oils, use your carrier oil and drop 4 tsps. into the container.
6. Place the lid on the storage container and roll the container between your hands a couple of times, then rotate the bottle using your first finger and thumb in an up and down motion.
7. This will help the oils to blend properly.

To apply:
Ensure that you are not allergic to any of the ingredients found in this recipe. When you are having problems with scoring you need to rub the remedy into your shoulders, upper chest, back of the neck and down your back prior to going to bed. This should relieve the snoring and help you to breathe better.

Prior to Shaving

Supplies that you will need:

Sweet Bay Essential Oils

Flaxseed Essential Oil

Geranium Essential Oil

Glass container with a sealable lid

Glass dram for blending with a pour spout

Directions for blending:
1. In order to prepare this blend properly, you will need to have a glass dram to use for preparation prior to placing it in the roller bottle. Using the oils start with the flaxseed oil and drop 20 drops into the dram.
2. Then, drop 2 drops of Geranium and 1 drop of Sweet Bay into the dram.
3. Roll the dram in the palms of your hands to blend the oils together.
4. Then, pour into your storage container that is glass.
5. Place the lid on the storage container and roll the container between your hands a couple of times, then rotate the bottle using your first finger and thumb in an up and down motion.
6. This will help the oils to blend properly.

To apply:

Ensure that you are not allergic to any of the ingredients found in this recipe. Prior to shaving in the morning apply this oil blend to your face to ensure a smooth shave. This will also help with soothing the face after you have shaved.

Chapter 11: Easy to follow recipes for home care needs

Disinfect your Room

Supplies that you will need:

Eucalyptus Essential Oils

Tea Tree Essential Oil

Thyme Essential Oil

Purified water

Glass Cleaner spray bottle

Glass dram for blending with a pour spout

Directions for blending:
1. In order to prepare this blend properly, you will need to have a glass dram to use for preparation prior to placing it in the roller bottle. Using the oils start with the Tea Tree Oil and drop 65 drops into the dram.
2. The use the Thyme Oil and drop in 50 drops into the dram.
3. Next, add in the Eucalyptus Oil in 35 drops into the dram.
4. Roll the dram in the palms of your hands to blend the oils together.
5. Then, pour into your glass house cleaner spray bottle.

6. Once you have poured in your blended Essential oils, use your 4 fluid ounces of purified water to fill the bottle.
7. Place the spray lid on the bottle and roll the ball between your hands a couple of times, then rotate the bottle using your first finger and thumb in an up and down motion.
8. This will help the oils to blend properly.

To apply:
This spray can be used multiple ways within your home. You can use it to disinfect your bathroom, your kitchen, your carpets and other appliances within your home. This is a great disinfectant to have on hand and is sure to smell delicious.

Air Freshener Disinfectant

Supplies that you will need:

Peppermint Essential Oil

Rosemary Essential Oil

Glass Spray Bottles

Purified Water

Glass dram for blending with a pour spout

Directions for blending:
1. In order to prepare this blend properly, you will need to have a glass dram to use for preparation prior to placing it in the glass spray bottle. Using the oils start with the Rosemary Oil and drop 56 drops into the dram.
2. The use the Peppermint Oil and drop in 36 drops.
3. Roll the dram in the palms of your hands to blend the oils together.
4. Then, pour into your spray glass bottle.
5. Once you have poured in your blended Essential oils, pour 4 fluid ounces of Purified water into the bottle.
6. Place the lid on the spray bottle and roll the bottle between your hands a couple of times, then rotate the bottle using your first finger and thumb in an up and down motion.
7. This will help the oils to blend properly.

To apply:

By mixing the ingredients you can start to disinfect your house with the antibacterial and antimicrobial power of Rosemary and Peppermint adds a touch of minty freshness. This spray is amazing in your home as a deodorizer as well as a germ fighter.

Stress Reduction

Supplies that you will need:

Cinnamon Essential Oil

Fennel Essential Oil

Chamomile Essential Oil

Diffuser

Purified Water

Glass dram for blending with a pour spout

Directions for blending:
1. In order to prepare this blend properly, you will need to have a glass dram to use for preparation prior to placing it in the glass spray bottle. Using the oils start with the Chamomile Oil and drop 9 drops into the dram.
2. Then, use the Cinnamon Oil and drop in 6 drops in the dram.
3. Next, place 5 drops of Fennel Oil in the dram.
4. Roll the dram in the palms of your hands to blend the oils together.
5. Once you have poured in your blended Essential oils, pour 4 fluid ounces of Purified water into the diffuser and add the oils.
6. Turn your diffuser on and sit back and enjoy the aroma.

To apply:

Start with mixing your oils together and then pour the purified water into your favorite diffuser. Once the water is in the diffuser pour in your oil blend and turn on the diffuser. Then sit back and enjoy the benefits of the oils.

Elevate Your Mood

Supplies that you will need:

Orange Essential Oil

Bergamot Essential Oil

Allspice Essential Oil

Geranium Essential Oil

Purified Water

Diffuser

Glass dram for blending with a pour spout

Directions for blending:
1. In order to prepare this blend properly, you will need to have a glass dram to use for preparation prior to placing it in the glass spray bottle. Using the oils start with the Geranium Oil and drop 5 drops into the dram.
2. Then, use the Bergamot Oil and drop in 4 drops.
3. Next, pour some Orange Oil, and Allspice Oil into the dram. You will need 3 drops.
4. Roll the dram in the palms of your hands to blend the oils together.
5. Once you have poured in your blended Essential oils, place the 4 fluid ounces of water into the diffuser and pour in the oil blend.
6. Turn on your diffuser and let the oil do its magic.

To apply:

This blend will increase your mood and also help you to elevate the moods of others in the same vicinity. Bergamot is known as a natural anti-depressant. This can increase the moods of children as well as those that suffer from depression.

Chapter 12: Easy to follow recipes for specific needs

Soothe those Aching Muscles

Supplies that you will need:

Ylang-Ylang Essential Oils

Spearmint Essential Oil

Lavender Essential Oil

Geranium Essential Oils

Glass bowl with sealable lid for storage

Your favorite carrier oils (grapeseed, hazelnut, sweet almond, or sesame)

Glass dram for blending with a pour spout

Directions for blending:
1. In order to prepare this blend properly, you will need to have a glass dram to use for preparation prior to placing it in the sealable glass jar for later use. Using the oils start with the Geranium and drop 5 drops into the dram.
2. Then, use the Spearmint, and Ylang-Ylang to drop in 4 drops each.
3. Next, add in the Lavender with 2 drops.
4. Roll the dram in the palms of your hands to blend the oils together.

5. Then, pour into your glass sealable container for storage.
6. Once you have poured in your blended Essential oils, use your carrier oil and fill the remaining space with the oil.
7. Place the lid on the storage container and roll the ball between your hands a couple of times, then rotate the bottle using your first finger and thumb in an up and down motion.
8. This will help the oils to blend properly.

To apply:

Verify that you are not allergic to any of the ingredients in this ointment prior to use. Then heat up some water to a temperature that is warm but not too hot. Then pour in the oils to a consistency that is okay for your skin. Place your hands in the basin of water and oil and let them soak for 20-30 minutes. This should relieve the muscles within your hands. This can also be applied to a bath and you can soak your body into the bath with warm water for 20-30 minutes to relieve the achy muscles from working long hours.

Strengthen your Plants as well as Repel Insects

Supplies that you will need:

Clove Essential Oils

Sage Essential Oil

Glass bowl with sealable lid for storage

Water

Glass dram for blending with a pour spout

Directions for blending:
1. In order to prepare this blend properly, you will need to have a glass dram to use for preparation prior to placing it in the sealable glass jar for later use. Using the oils start with the Sage Oil and drop 10 drops into the dram.
2. Then, use the Clove Oil to drop in 5 drops each.
3. Roll the dram in the palms of your hands to blend the oils together.
4. Once you have poured in your blended Essential oils, use the water to fill the pitcher and place the oil blend into the pitcher

To apply:

Use the pitcher to hydrate and replenish the plants within your garden by mixing the oils and then blend them properly. Once blended pour into a pitcher of water. This recipe can be used daily.

Calm Down Fido

Supplies that you will need:

Chamomile Essential Oils

Mandarin Essential Oil

Lavender Essential Oil

Glass spray bottle

Purified Water

Glass dram for blending with a pour spout

Directions for blending:

1. In order to prepare this blend properly, you will need to have as glass dram to use for preparation prior to placing it in the sealable glass jar for later use. Start by pouring Chamomile and Lavender Oil drops into the dram. You will need 50 drops each.
2. Then, use the Mandarin Oil with 4 drops in the dram.
3. Roll the dram in the palms of your hands to blend the oils together.
4. Then, pour into your glass spray bottle.
5. Once you have poured in your blended Essential oils, use your purified water of 4 ounces to fill the bottle.
6. Place the sprayer nozzle on the bottle and roll the bottle between your hands a couple of times, then rotate the bottle using your first finger and thumb in an up and down motion.

7. This will help the oils to blend properly.

To apply:

Verify that you are not allergic to any of the ingredients in this ointment prior to use. The combination of Chamomile, lavender, and Mandarin combined in a spray bottle will help calm your pets and give them a sedated state. This works well with overactive pets. This would be great for those puppy stages.

Chapter 13: Easy to follow recipes for use in spas and beauty centers

Facial for Problem Skin

Supplies that you will need:
Bois De rose Essential Oils
Myrrh Essential Oil
Lavender Essential Oil
Chamomile Essential Oil
Kukui Nut Oil
Glass dram for blending with a pour spout

Directions for blending:
1. In order to prepare this blend properly, you will need to have a glass dram to use for preparation prior to placing it in the roller bottle. Using the oils start with the Chamomile and Myrrh Oil. You will need 3 drops placed into the dram.
2. Then, pour the Bois De Rose as well as, the Lavender Oil into the dram with 5 drops per oil.
3. Roll the dram in the palms of your hands to blend the oils together.
4. Then, pour into your glass storage container.

5. Once you have poured in your blended Essential oils, use your Kukui Nut oil to fill with 2 tablespoons.
6. Place lid on the storage container and roll the container between your hands a couple of times, then rotate the bottle using your first finger and thumb in an up and down motion.
7. This will help the oils to blend properly.

To apply:

Verify that you are not allergic to the ingredients in this facial ointment. Wash your face prior to use and then apply the oils to your face for a wonderful and refreshing facial. The lavender will rejuvenate the skin and the Myrrh and Chamomile are replenishing and refreshing.

Hair Growth Formula

Supplies that you will need:
Clary Sage Essential Oils
Rosemary Essential Oil
Lavender Essential Oil
Peppermint Oil
Apricot Essential Oil
Coconut Oil
Castor Oil
Glass storage container that is sealable
Glass dram for blending with a pour spout

Directions for blending:
1. In order to prepare this blend properly, you will need to have a glass dram to use for preparation prior to placing it in the roller bottle. Using the oils, start with the Rosemary Oil. You will need 12 drops placed into the dram.
2. Then, pour the Lavender, Clary Sage, and Peppermint Oils into the dram with 6 drops per oil.
3. Next, you will need to add in the 1 ounce of Apricot oil, Castor Oil, and 2 ounces of Coconut Oil into the dram.

4. Roll the dram in the palms of your hands to blend the oils together.
5. Then, pour into your glass storage container.
6. Place lid on the storage container and roll the container between your hands a couple of times, then rotate the bottle using your first finger and thumb in an up and down motion.
7. This will help the oils to blend properly.

To apply:
Verify that you are not allergic to the ingredients in this facial ointment. Place all the oils in the container and then blend them properly. Once blended you will need to apply to your hair and allow it to sit on your head for a couple of hours. This will induce hair growth.

Reduction of Stress

Supplies that you will need:
Allspice Essential Oil
Melissa Essential Oils
Purified Water
Glass dram for blending with a pour spout

Directions for blending:
1. In order to prepare this blend properly, you will need to have a glass dram to use for preparation prior to placing it in the roller bottle. Using the oils start with the Allspice and Melissa Oil and drop 10 drops into the dram.
2. Roll the dram in the palms of your hands to blend the oils together.
3. Pour in the purified water and then add your oil blend into the diffuser with the water.
4. Turn on the diffuser and enjoy.

To apply:
Pour the purified water into the diffuser and add in the essential oil blend. Then turn on the diffuser and enjoy the essential oils throughout your home. This will create a stress reduced environment.

Relief from Fatigue

Supplies that you will need:
Cumin Essential Oils
Lime Essential Oil
Clove Essential Oil
Your favorite carrier oils
Glass storage container
Glass dram for blending with a pour spout

Directions for blending:
1. In order to prepare this blend properly, you will need to have a glass dram to use for preparation prior to placing it in the roller bottle. Pour the Lime, Clove, and Cumin oil into the dram using 5 drops form each oil.
2. Roll the dram in the palms of your hands to blend the oils together.
3. Then, pour into your Storage container.
4. Once you have poured in your blended Essential oils, add in the carrier oil using 1 tablespoon of oil.
5. Place the lid on the storage container and roll the container between your hands a couple of times, then rotate the bottle using your first finger and thumb in an up and down motion.
6. This will help the oils to blend properly.

To apply:

Fatigue is difficult to combat but with this oil blend for massaging you will be able to combat the effects of fatigue by massaging the back of your neck, the chest, the shoulders, and then down the center of your back with the oil. This will help fee less fatigued and more easily alert.

Chapped Lips Roller Ball

Supplies that you will need:

Sandalwood Essential Oils

Macadamia Essential Oil

Lavender Essential Oil

Aloe Vera

Your 10-15 mL roller ball applicator

Your favorite carrier oils

Glass dram for blending with a pour spout

Directions for blending:
7. In order to prepare this blend properly, you will need to have a glass dram to use for preparation prior to placing it in the roller bottle. Using the oils start with the Lavender Oil and drop 3 drops into the dram.
8. The use the Sandalwood and drop in 2 drops.
9. Next, add in the macadamia in 1 tsp increment.
10. Roll the dram in the palms of your hands to blend the oils together.
11. Then, pour into your roller ball applicator.
12. Once you have poured in your blended Essential oils, use your carrier oil and fill the remaining space with the oil.
13. Place the lid on the roller ball and roll the ball between your hands a couple of times, then rotate the

bottle using your first finger and thumb in an up and down motion.
14. This will help the oils to blend properly.

To apply:

Apply the Aloe Vera to your lips prior to using this treatment for chapped lips. When using it on your child apply the roller ball to the lips and gently roll it across the bottom lip and then have them mush their lips together to spread the treatment. This will help to treat chapped lips and nourish the skin around the lips.

Repair Your Hair

Supplies that you will need:
Rosemary Essential Oils
Sweet Bay Essential Oil
Cedarwood Essential Oil
Geranium Essential Oil
Jojoba Oil
Glass storage container
Glass dram for blending with a pour spout

Directions for blending:
1. In order to prepare this blend properly, you will need to have a glass dram to use for preparation prior to placing it in the roller bottle. Using the oils start with the Cedarwood, Sweet Bay, and Rosemary Oil and drop 8 drops into the dram.
2. Then use the Geranium Oil in increments of 2 drops.
3. Roll the dram in the palms of your hands to blend the oils together.
4. Then, pour into your storage container.
5. Once you have poured in your blended Essential oils, add in the jojoba carrier oil so that you can blend the oils with the carrier.
6. Place the lid on the storage container and roll the container between your hands a couple of times, then

rotate the bottle using your first finger and thumb in an up and down motion.
7. This will help the oils to blend properly.

To apply:

When you mix the oils together and combine them with the jojoba oil you will be able to apply it to your hair and let it sit for several hours. Then once it has set for several hours you can wash your hair twice with an organic shampoo. This will clean out the oils left over. The oil blend will replenish the hair and restore it. You can use this oil as much as you like throughout the week until your hair is fully restored.

Chapter 14: Profiles that you must be aware of for each oil that you use.

Essential Oils have a specific profile that makes up their chemical compounds. When you are working with Essential Oils you will need to know thee profiles so that you can use them properly.

Below is a short list of the profiles for several of the oils mentioned in this book.

Antiseptic Essential Oils

Bergamot

Cedarwood

Clove

Chamomile

Eucalyptus

Jasmine

Juniper

Grapefruit

Ylang-Ylang

Orange

Sandalwood

Lavender

Patchouli
Myrrh
Lemon
Cinnamon
Rosemary
Thyme
Peppermint
Clary Sage

Antibiotic Essential Oils

Bergamot
Lavender
Lemon
Tea Tree
Geranium
Patchouli
Thyme
Clove
Eucalyptus
Cinnamon

Antifungal Essential Oil

Tea Tree

Patchouli

Eucalyptus

Cedarwood

Clove

Myrrh

Antiviral Essential Oil

Eucalyptus

Clove

Tea Tree

Cinnamon

Melissa

Thyme

Anti-infectious Essential Oil

Peppermint

Chamomile

Patchouli

Lemon

Clary Sage

Sandalwood

Palmarosa

Lavender

Eucalyptus

Thyme

Antibiotic is a term that is used to designate a chemical or Essential Oil compound that will prevent against infection and bacterial growths. These are used in the same way that the modern medical field would use antibiotic pills. When you take an antibiotic, you will be able to clear out any infections that have entered your body or skin. These can be used topically or through inhalation.

An antiseptic will destroy any microbes that have come in contact with your body and then prevents the development of the microbes so that they do not further bother your health.

Antifungals help to prevent fungal growths on your body. This includes the fungal growth on the toes and feet. By using an antifungal, you are able to prevent having fungal issues.

Antiviral Essential oils will prevent the growth of viral contaminants. This can be accomplished by using one of the antivirals in the list above or several of them. There are several more oils that can be included in the above profiles however I only included the ones that are listed within this book so that you had more information on the oils that you will be using.

Now that you have learned a bit about Essential Oils and their uses, you will be more prepared to help yourself and your family use Essential Oils to improve the health within your home.

Chapter 15: Easy to Follow Recipes for Ailments over 300 to Follow

For each recipe, you will need a dram that is made of glass to mix them in. Then, you will need to follow proper blending procedures to ensure that the blending is done properly. Next, you will need to apply your carrier oil or purified water if it calls for either. Many of these recipes will be used through topical, diffuser, inhalation, or in a soaking foot bath or bathtub.

These recipes will read in this format:
- Name of the blend
- Oils needed with incremental
- Supplies needed

Common Ailments

Most of the blends listed below can be used as a massage oil on the area that needs treatment as well as a bath or foot soak. They can be used on a regular basis or whenever necessary. These recipes are simple to follow. Some of them provide ingredients that are needed and allow you to gauge the aroma effect by judging your own number of drops needed. While some provide you an exact number of drops needed which is located within the () section, remember that all oils need to be tested prior to using and should be diluted to the proper %.

Sleep Ready

Supplies that you will need:

Chamomile (Roman) Essence Oil (2)

Lavender Essence Oils (3)

Vetiver Essence Oils (2)

Rollerball Applicator 10ml

Blending Glass Dram

Carrier oils that you like

Breathing Is Easy

Supplies that you will need:

Tea Tree Essence Oil (1)

Rosemary Essence Oils (1)

Eucalyptus Essence Oils (1)

Cardamom Essence Oil (1)

Lemon Essence Oil (1)

Peppermint Essence Oil (2)

Rollerball Applicator 10ml

Blending Glass Dram

Carrier oils that you like

Insect Itch Spray

Supplies that you will need:

Juniper Berries Essence Oil (2)

Tea Tree Essence Oils (2)

Lemon Essence Oils (1)

Borage Essence Oil (1tsp)
Spray Bottle - glass
Rollerball Applicator 10ml
Blending Glass Dram
Carrier oils that you like

Lice No More

Supplies that you will need:
Peppermint Essence Oil (5)
Ginger Essence Oils (5)
Lavender Essence Oils (5)
Walnut Essence Oil (1tsp)
Rollerball Applicator 10ml
Blending Glass Dram
Carrier oils that you like
Glass Storage

Bath Relief for PMS

Supplies that you will need:
Geranium Essence Oil (5)
Bergamot Essence Oils (5)
Palmarosa Essence Oil (5)
Rollerball Applicator 10ml
Blending Glass Dram
Carrier oils that you like

Female Deodorant

Supplies that you will need:

Jojoba Oil

Lavender Essence Oils (2)

Cornstarch

Tolu Balsam (3)

Rollerball Applicator 10ml

Blending Glass Dram

Carrier oils that you like

Glass Container

Oily Hair No More

Supplies that you will need:

Rosemary Essence Oil (8)

Grapeseed Oils (2tsp)

Ylang-Ylang Essence Oils (9)

Lime Essence Oil (9)

Spray Bottle - glass

Blending Glass Dram

Carrier oils that you like

Cellulite Begone

Supplies that you will need:

Benzoin Essence Oil (5)

Lemon Essence Oils (5)

Rosemary Essence Oil (5)

Fennel Essence Oil (5)

Glass container with a sealable lid

Blending Glass Dram

Carrier oils that you like

Muscles Heal

Supplies that you will need:

Rosemary Essence Oil (2)

Nutmeg Essence Oils (3)

Ginger Essence Oil (5)

Ylang-Ylang Essence Oil (5)

Glass container with a sealable lid

Blending Glass Dram

Carrier oils that you like

Increase My Strength

Supplies that you will need:

Peppermint Essence Oils (5)

Grapefruit Essence Oil (5)

Ginger Essence Oil (6)

Lemon Essence Oil (4)

Thyme Essence Oil (5)

Celery Essence Oil (5)

Storage Container - glass

Grapeseed Oil (2tbsp)

Blending Glass Dram

Carrier oils that you like

Snore No More

Supplies that you will need:
Cajeput Essence Oil (4)

Lavender Essence Oils (3)

Myrtle Essence Oil (4)

Chamomile Essence Oil (3)

Marjoram Essence Oil (3)

Petitgrain Essence Oil (3)

Container - glass

Blending Glass Dram

Carrier oils that you like

Before You Shave

Supplies that you will need:
Geranium Essence Oil (2)

Sweet Bay Essence Oils (1)

Flaxseed Essence Oil (20)

Container - glass

Blending Glass Dram

No More Germs

Supplies that you will need:
Purified Water (4 fl. oz.)

Eucalyptus Essence Oils (35)

Thyme Essence Oil (50)
Tea Tree Essence Oil (65)
Glass Spray Bottle
Blending Glass Dram
Carrier oils that you like

Air Smells Good

Supplies that you will need:
Purified Water (4 fl. oz.)
Rosemary Essence Oil (56)
Peppermint Essence Oil (36)
Spray Bottles - glass
Blending Glass Dram

No More Stress #1

Supplies that you will need:
Chamomile Essence Oil (9)
Cinnamon Essence Oil (6)
Fennel Essence Oil (5)
Purified Water
Diffuser
Blending Glass Dram

No More Stress #2

Supplies that you will need:
Melissa Essence Oils (10)

Allspice Essence Oil (10)

Purified Water

Blending Glass Dram

Lift Me Up

Supplies that you will need:

Purified Water (4 fl. oz.)

Allspice Essence Oil (3)

Orange Essence Oil (3)

Geranium Essence Oil (5)

Bergamot Essence Oil (4)

Diffuser

Blending Glass Dram

Ache Begone

Supplies that you will need:

Geranium Essence Oils (5)

Ylang-Ylang Essence Oils (4)

Lavender Essence Oil (2)

Spearmint Essence Oil (4)

Carrier oils that you like

*(grapeseed, sweet almond, hazelnut, or sesame)

Container - glass

Blending Glass Dram

Plant Growth

Supplies that you will need:

Container - glass
Sage Essence Oil (10)
Clove Essence Oils (5)
Water (4 fl. oz.)
Blending Glass Dram

Doggy Sit Still

Supplies that you will need:

Chamomile Essence Oils (50)
Mandarin Essence Oil (4)
Lavender Essence Oil (50)
Spray Bottle - glass
Purified Water (4 fl. oz.)
Blending Glass Dram

Clear My Skin

Supplies that you will need:

Bois De Rose Essence Oils (5)
Kukui Nut Oil (2tbsp)
Myrrh Essence Oil (3)
Chamomile Essence Oil (3)
Lavender Essence Oil (5)
Blending Glass Dram

Grow More Hair

Supplies that you will need:

Peppermint Oil (6)

Clary Sage Essence Oils (6)

Lavender Essence Oil (6)

Rosemary Essence Oil (12)

Castor Oil (2-oz)

Apricot Essence Oil (2-oz)

Coconut Oil (2-oz)

Container - glass

Blending Glass Dram

Fatigue Relief

Supplies that you will need:

Cumin Essence Oils (5)

Lime Essence Oil (5)

Clove Essence Oil (5)

Carrier oils that you like

Container - glass

Blending Glass Dram

ChapStick for Lips

Supplies that you will need:

Aloe Vera

Sandalwood Essence Oils (2)

Lavender Essence Oil (3)

Macadamia Essence Oil (1tsp)
Rollerball Applicator 10ml
Carrier oils you like
Blending Glass Dram

Hair Repair

Supplies that you will need:

Jojoba Oil (4 fl. oz.)
Sweet Bay Essence Oil (8)
Rosemary Essence Oils (8)
Geranium Essence Oil (2)
Cedarwood Essence Oil (8)
Glass Container
Blending Glass Dram

Stress Is Gone

Supplies that you will need:

Clary Sage Essence Oil (3)
Purified Water
Lavender Essence Oil (1)
Lemon Bark Essence Oil (1)
Blending Glass Dram

Stress Relief Finally

Supplies that you will need:

Purified Water

Vetiver Essence Oil (1)
Lavender Essence Oil (2)
Chamomile (Roman) Essence Oil (2)
Blending Glass Dram

Reduce That Stress
Supplies that you will need:
Purified Water
Melissa Essence Oils (10)
Allspice Essence Oil (10)
Blending Glass Dram

Anxiety Begone
Supplies that you will need:
Purified Water
Clary Sage Essence oil (2)
Patchouli Essence Oil (1)
Geranium Essence Oil (2)
Ylang-Ylang Essence Oil (1)
Blending Glass Dram

Calm the Anxious
Supplies that you will need:
Purified Water
Ylang-Ylang Essence Oil (1)
Patchouli Essence Oil (1)

Cedarwood Essence Oil (2)

Wild Orange Essence Oil (2)

Blending Glass Dram

Happily Wake Up

Supplies that you will need:

Purified Water

Bergamot Essence Oil (3)

Ylang-Ylang Essence Oil (3)

Blending Glass Dram

Mood Goes up on a Tuesday

Supplies that you will need:

Purified Water

Diffuser

Allspice Essence Oil (3)

Geranium Essence Oil (5)

Bergamot Essence Oil (4)

Orange Essence Oil (3)

Blending Glass Dram

Lift My Mood, Now

Supplies that you will need:

Clove Essence Oil (2)

Patchouli Essence Oils (4)

Rose Essence Oil (5)

Geranium Essence Oil (4)

Blending Glass Dram

Container - glass

Carrier oil of your choice

Smell Those Mountains

Supplies that you will need:
Purified Water

Idaho Balsam Fir Essence Oil (3)

Ylang-Ylang Essence Oil (3)

Blending Glass Dram

Boosting Your Energy #1

Supplies that you will need:
Purified Water

Lemon Essence Oil (2)

Frankincense Essence Oil (2)

Peppermint Essence Oil (2)

Blending Glass Dram

Boosting Your Energy #2

Supplies that you will need:
Purified Water

Black Pepper Essence Oil (3)

Rosemary Essence Oil (3)

Blending Glass Dram

Boosting Your Energy #3

Supplies that you will need:

Purified Water

Sweet Orange Essence oil (5)

Lemon Essence Oil (5)

Grapefruit Essence Oil (5)

Cinnamon Bark Essence Oil (2)

Blending Glass Dram

Menopause No More #1

Supplies that you will need:

Purified Water

Rosemary Essence Oil (20)

Peppermint Essence Oil (10)

Ylang-Ylang Essence Oil (10)

Chamomile (Roman) Essence Oil (10)

Rose Otto Essence Oil (10)

Geranium Essence Oil (20)

Lavender Essence Oil (20)

Blending Glass Dram

Menopause No More #2

Supplies that you will need:

Purified Water

Aloe Vera Gel (1tsp)

Peppermint Essence Oil (5)

Lavender Essence Oil (5)

Blending Glass Dram

Spray Bottle - glass

Menopause No More #3

Supplies that you will need:

Ylang-Ylang Essence Oil (5)

Bergamot Essence Oil (5)

Clary Sage Essence Oil (10)

Sandalwood Essence Oil (5)

Rose Otto Essence Oil (10)

Geranium Essence Oil (5)

Coconut Oil - Fractionated (1tsp)

Blending Glass Dram

Rollerball 10 ml-glass

Cramps from PMS

Supplies that you will need:

Clary Sage Essence Oil (3)

Geranium Essence Oil (1)

Lavender Essence Oil (2)

Avocado oil (2tsp)

Blending Glass Dram

Rollerball 10 ml-glass

Relieve My PMS
Supplies that you will need:
Jojoba (2tbsp)
Cypress Essence Oil (4)
Peppermint Essence Oil (5)
Lavender Essence Oil (3)
Blending Glass Dram
Roller Ball - glass

Premenstrual Relief of Symptoms
Supplies that you will need:
Peppermint Essence Oil (10)
Lavender Essence Oil (10)
Lemon Essence Oil (10)
Whole Milk
Epsom Salt
Blending Glass Dram

Headache Relief
Supplies that you will need:
Purified Water
Peppermint Essence Oil (2)
Lavender Essence Oil (2)
Rosemary Essence Oil (1)
Eucalyptus Essence Oil (1)
Blending Glass Dram

Stress Headache

Supplies that you will need:

Purified Water

Peppermint Essence Oil (2)

Sweet Marjoram Essence oil (2)

Lavender Essence Oil (2)

Rosemary Essence Oil (2)

Thyme Essence Oil (2)

Blending Glass Dram

Sinus Cavity Headache

Supplies that you will need:

Purified Water

Frankincense Essence Oil (2)

Basil Essence Oil (2)

Lavender Essence oil (4)

Peppermint Essence Oil (4)

Blending Glass Dram

No More Sickness

Supplies that you will need:

Purified Water

Spearmint Essence Oil (1)

Grapefruit Essence Oil (1)

Sweet Orange Essence oil (1)

Lime Essence Oil (1)

Blending Glass Dram

Anti-Nausea Oil Blend

Supplies that you will need:

Carrier Oil (30ml) whatever you choose

Peppermint Essence Oil (5)

Lavender Essence Oil (5)

Blending Glass Dram

Sickness Go Away

Supplies that you will need:

Peppermint Essence Oil (5)

Lemon Essence Oil *(3)

Blending Glass Dram

Carrier Oil (30ml) - your choice

Ginger Blocks This Nausea

Supplies that you will need:

Peppermint Essence Oil (10)

Ginger Essence Oil (10)

Chamomile Essence Oil (10)

Blending Glass Dram

Carrier Oil (30ml) - your choice

Grow Me Some Hair

Supplies that you will need:

Castor Oil Jamaican Black (0.25 cups)

Cedarwood Essence Oil (10)

Peppermint Bark Essence Oil (10)

Lavender Essence Oil (10)

Blending Glass Dram

Rosemary Essence Oil (10)

Coconut Oil (0.25 cups)

Perfectly Clean Face

Supplies that you will need:

Jasmine Essence Oil (10)

Hazelnut carrier Oil (2tbsp)

Rose Essence Oil (10)

Frankincense Essence Oil (10)

Blending Glass Dram

Oily Skin Facial

Supplies that you will need:

Grapeseed Carrier Oil (2tbsp)

Petitgrain Essence Oil (10)

Orange Essence Oil (10)

Lemon Essence Oil (10)

Blending Glass Dram

Acne Clear Skin Facial

Supplies that you will need:

Kukui Nut Carrier Oil (2 tbsp)
Bois De Rose Essence Oil (5)
Chamomile Essence Oil (10)
Lavender Essence Oil (5)
Myrrh Essence Oil (10)
Blending Glass Dram

Repel the Bug

Supplies that you will need:
Lemongrass Essence Oil (3)
Citronella Essence Oil (3)
Blending Glass Dram

Bronchitis Is Gone

Supplies that you will need:
Clove Essence Oil (2)
Myrrh Essence Oil (2)
Ravensara Essence Oil (6)
Frankincense Essence Oil (15)
Sage Essence Oil (2)
Blending Glass Dram
Carrier oil (30ml) - your choice

Influenza No-No

Supplies that you will need:
Purified Water

Clove Essence Oil (4)

Oregano Essence Oil (8)

Hyssop Essence Oil (5)

Ravensara Essence Oil (10)

Cinnamon Leaf Essence Oil (7)

Thyme Essence Oil (6)

Blending Glass Dram

Pneumonia No More

Supplies that you will need:

Oregano Essence Oil (2)

Ravensara Essence Oil (8)

Peppermint Essence Oil (2)

Rosemary Essence Oil (10)

Frankincense Essence Oil (8)

Blending Glass Dram

Rollerball - glass

Carrier Oil (30ml) - your choice

Balanced at Home

Supplies that you will need:

Purified Water

Bergamot Essence Oil (2)

Juniper Berry Essence Oil (1)

Lavender Essence Oil (2)

Blending Glass Dram

Breeze of the Sea

Supplies that you will need:

Purified Water

Tangerine Essence Oil (3)

Arborvitae Essence Oil (2)

Cypress Essence Oil (3)

Blending Glass Dram

Clean and Fresh Air

Supplies that you will need:

Purified Water

Lavender Essence Oil (3)

Tangerine Essence Oil (3)

Eucalyptus Essence Oil (2)

Blending Glass Dram

Welcome Home Scent

Supplies that you will need:

Purified Water

Lemon Essence Oil (3)

Orange Essence Oil (3)

Cinnamon Essence Oil (3)

Blending Glass Dram

Home Is Delightful

Supplies that you will need:

Purified Water

Lime Essence Oil (3)

Tea Tree Essence Oil (2)

Spearmint Essence Oil (2)

Blending Glass Dram

Pumpkin Spice Latte

Supplies that you will need:

Purified Water

Thieves Essence Oil (3)

Orange Essence Oil (3)

Blending Glass Dram

Apple Holiday

Supplies that you will need:

Purified Water

Orange Essence Oil (4)

Ginger Essence Oil (2)

Cinnamon Essence Oil (2)

Blending Glass Dram

Christmas Frazier

Supplies that you will need:

Purified Water

Blue Spruce Idaho Essence Oil (2)

Pine Essence Oil (2)

Balsam Fir Idaho Essence Oil (2)

Blending Glass Dram

Kids Are Out like Babies

Supplies that you will need:

Purified Water

Cedarwood Essence Oil (3)

Orange Essence Oil (3)

Blending Glass Dram

Dreams Begone

Supplies that you will need:

Purified Water

Hawaiian Sandalwood Essence Oil (5)

Lavender Essence Oil (5)

Vetiver Essence Oil (3)

Ylang-Ylang Essence Oil (3)

Rose Essence Oil (4)

Bergamot Essence Oil (5)

Tangerine Essence Oil (6)

Juniper Essence Oil (3)

Blending Glass Dram

Focus and Concentrate

Supplies that you will need:

Purified Water

Lemon Essence Oil (4)

Rosemary Essence Oil (4)

Blending Glass Dram

Comfort

Supplies that you will need:

Lavender Essence Oil (4)

Mandarin Essence Oil (3)

Chamomile (Roman) (2)

Carrier Oil (30ml) - your choice

Blending Glass Dram

Breathe Better

Supplies that you will need:

Lemon Essence Oil (2)

Rosemary Essence Oil (5)

Eucalyptus Essence Oil (5)

Peppermint Essence Oil (3)

Blending Glass Dram

Carrier Oil (30ml) - your choice

Depression Blocker

Supplies that you will need:

Mandarin Essence Oil (4)

Neroli Essence Oil (4)

Blending Glass Dram

Carrier Oil (30ml) - your choice

Support for the Family

Supplies that you will need:

Purified Water

Lavender Essence Oil (7)

Rose Essence Oil (3)

Mandarin Essence Oil (10)

Blending Glass Dram

Massage for Infants

Supplies that you will need:

Lavender Essence Oil (2)

Chamomile (Roman) Essence Oil (1)

Blending Glass Dram

Carrier oil (30ml) - Jojoba, Kukui, or Sweet Almond

Child's Massage

Supplies that you will need:

Lavender Essence Oil (2)

Chamomile (Roman) Essence Oil (1)

Mandarin Essence Oil (3)

Blending Glass Dram

Carrier Oil (30ml) - Jojoba, Kukui, Sweet Almond

Stretch Marks Begone

Supplies that you will need:

Frankincense Essence Oil (7)

Neroli Essence Oil (3)

Blending Glass Dram

Carrier Oil (30ml) - your choice

Back Pain Begone

Supplies that you will need:

Lavender Essence Oil (7)

Chamomile (Roman) Essence Oil (3)

Blending Glass Dram

Carrier Oil (30ml) - your choice

Reduce the Pain

Supplies that you will need:

Carrier Oil (30ml) - your choice

Lavender Essence Oil (5)

Frankincense Essence Oil (5)

Blending Glass Dram

Anxiety Is Not My Problem

Supplies that you will need:

Vetiver Essence Oil (2)

Rose Essence Oil (3)

Mandarin Essence Oils (5)

Blending Glass Dram

Carrier Oil (30ml) - your choice

Reflexology for Digestive Help

Supplies that you will need:

Purified Water

Fennel Essence Oil (4)

Lavender Essence Oil (3)

Peppermint Essence Oil (3)

Blending Glass Dram

Carrier Oil (30ml) - your choice

Constipation Blend for Massages

Supplies that you will need:

Sweet Fennel Essence Oil (3)

Cardamom Essence Oil (4)

Lemon Essence Oil (4)

Lavender Essence Oil (7)

Blending Glass Dram

Apricot Kernel Oil (30ml)

Premenstrual Massage

Supplies that you will need:

Apricot Kernel (30ml)

Geranium Essence Oil (6)

Lavender Essence Oil (14)

Clary Sage Essence Oil (6)

Bergamot Essence Oil (10)

Blending Glass Dram

Foot Cream for Massaging

Supplies that you will need:

Lavender Essence Oil (10)

Peppermint Essence Oil (7)

Blending Glass Dram

Cream (2-oz)

Foot Massage

Supplies that you will need:

Juniper berry Essence Oil (6)

Bay Laurel Essence Oil (4)

Grapefruit Essence Oil (8)

Blending Glass Dram

Apricot Kernel (30ml)

Organic Sunflower (30ml)

Poor Circulation

Supplies that you will need:

Black Pepper Essence Oil (6)

Rosemary Essence Oil (5)

Lemon Essence Oil (7)

Blending Glass Dram

Apricot Kernel (30ml)

Home Synergy

Supplies that you will need:

Lavender Essence Oil (20)

Rose Geranium Essence Oil (7)

Tangerine Essence Oil (18)

Vetiver Essence Oil (5)

Blending Glass Dram

Carrier Oil (30ml) - your choice

Anxiety Massage

Supplies that you will need:

Sandalwood Essence Oil (4)

Tangerine Essence Oil (7)

Vetiver Essence Oils (2)

Rose Essence Oils (2)

Blending Glass Dram

Carrier Oil (30ml) - your choice

Carpal Tunnel

Supplies that you will need:

Peppermint Essence Oil (4)

Juniper berry Essence Oil (7)

Lemon Essence Oil (8)

Lavender Essence Oil (11)

Blending Glass Dram
Arnica Herbal Oils (10%)
Apricot Kernel Oil (80%)
St. John's Wort Herbal (10%)

Pain Gel

Supplies that you will need:
Peppermint Essence Oil (11)
Birch Essence Oil (8)
Bay Laurel Essence Oil (14)
Lavender Essence Oil (27)
Blending Glass Dram
Aloe Vera Gel

Bursitis

Supplies that you will need:
Birch Essence Oil (4)
Cypress Essence Oil (4)
Eucalyptus Essence Oil (3)
Juniper Berry Essence Oil (2)
Chamomile (German) Essence Oil (5)
Cardamom Essence Oil (4)
Helichrysum Essence Oil (6)
Peppermint Essence Oil (2)
Lavender Essence Oil (6)
Rosemary Essence Oil (4)

Lemon Essence Oil (3)
Blending Glass Dram
St. John's Wort
Arnica Oil

Sprains

Supplies that you will need:
Black Pepper Essence Oil
Grapefruit Essence Oil
Lemon Essence Oil
Sweet Marjoram Essence Oil
Birch Essence Oil
Chamomile (Roman) Essence Oil
Clove Bud Essence Oil
Peppermint Essence Oil
Lemongrass Essence Oil
Juniper Berry Essence Oil
Lavender Essence Oil
Laurel Essence Oil
Cypress Essence Oil
Helichrysum Essence Oil
Eucalyptus Essence Oil
Cardamom Essence Oil
Chamomile (German) Essence Oil
Spearmint Essence Oil
Blending Glass Dram

St. John's Wort

Arnica

This would be measured based on your olfactory senses and what you find attractive to smell.

Plantar Fasciitis

Supplies that you will need:

Purified Water

Eucalyptus Essence Oil

Cardamom Essence Oil

Lavender Essence Oil

Spearmint Essence Oil

Birch Essence Oil

Chamomile (German) Essence Oil

Sweet Marjoram Essence Oil

Clary Sage Essence Oil

Chamomile (Roman) Essence Oil

Clove Bud Essence Oil

Helichrysum Essence Oil

Peppermint Essence Oil

Rosemary Essence Oil

Laurel Essence Oil

Blending Glass Dram

Arnica

St. John's Wort

Apply to a foot bath

Whiplash

Supplies that you will need:

Cardamom Essence Oil

Helichrysum Essence Oil

Petitgrain Essence Oil

Juniper Berry Essence Oil

Frankincense Essence Oil

Chamomile (Roman) Essence Oil

Birch Essence Oil

Clove Bud Essence Oil

Black Pepper Essence Oil

Neroli Essence Oil

Sweet Marjoram Essence Oil

Cypress Essence Oil

Rosemary Essence Oil

Chamomile (German) Essence Oil

Peppermint Essence Oil

Clary Sage Essence Oil

Spearmint Essence Oil

Lavender Essence Oil

Laurel Essence Oil

Vetiver Essence Oil

Blending Glass Dram

St. John's Wort

Arnica

Massage into skin

Sciatica

Supplies that you will need:
Cardamom Essence Oil

Helichrysum Essence Oil

Petitgrain Essence Oil

Juniper Berry Essence Oil

Frankincense Essence Oil

Chamomile (Roman) Essence Oil

Birch Essence Oil

Clove Bud Essence Oil

Neroli Essence Oil

Sweet Marjoram Essence Oil

Cypress Essence Oil

Rosemary Essence Oil

Chamomile (German) Essence Oil

Peppermint Essence Oil

Clary Sage Essence Oil

Spearmint Essence Oil

Lavender Essence Oil

Laurel Essence Oil

Cinnamon Leaf Essence Oil

Blending Glass Dram

St. John's Wort

Arnica

Massage into skin

Spasms

Supplies that you will need:

Petitgrain Essence Oil

Juniper Berry Essence Oil

Birch Essence Oil

Sweet Marjoram Essence Oil

Cypress Essence Oil

Chamomile (German) Essence Oil

Peppermint Essence Oil

Clary Sage Essence Oil

Spearmint Essence Oil

Lavender Essence Oil

Fennel Essence Oil

Lemon Essence Oil

Blending Glass dram

St. John's Wort

Arnica

Massage into skin

Fibromyalgia

Supplies that you will need:

Angelic Root Essence Oil

Helichrysum Essence Oil

Ylang Ylang Essence Oil

Ginger Essence Oil

Ravensara Essence Oil

Chamomile (Roman) Essence Oil

Birch Essence Oil

Mandarin Essence Oil

Neroli Essence Oil

Sweet Marjoram Essence Oil

Sandalwood Essence Oil

Rosemary Essence Oil

Chamomile (German) Essence Oil

Rose Essence Oil

Vetiver Essence Oil

Spearmint Essence Oil

Black Pepper Essence Oil

Laurel Essence Oil

Blending Glass Dram

St. John's Wort

Arnica

Massage into skin

Osteoarthritis

Supplies that you will need:

Helichrysum Essence Oil

Juniper Berry Essence Oil

Birch Essence Oil

Clove Bud Essence Oil

Sweet Marjoram Essence Oil

Cypress Essence Oil

Rosemary Essence Oil

Chamomile (German) Essence Oil

Peppermint Essence Oil

Grapefruit Essence Oil

Spearmint Essence Oil

Lavender Essence Oil

Laurel Essence Oil

Palmarosa Essence Oil

Blending Glass Dram

Massage into skin

Rheumatoid

Supplies that you will need:

Grapefruit Essence Oil

Helichrysum Essence Oil

Ginger Essence Oil

Juniper Berry Essence Oil

Frankincense Essence Oil

Chamomile (Roman) Essence Oil

Birch Essence Oil

Clove Bud Essence Oil

Black Pepper Essence Oil

Sweet Marjoram Essence Oil

Cypress Essence Oil

Rosemary Essence Oil

Chamomile (German) Essence Oil

Peppermint Essence Oil

Rose Essence Oil

Spearmint Essence Oil

Lavender Essence Oil

Laurel Essence Oil

Vetiver Essence Oil

Thyme Essence Oils

Ylang Ylang Essence Oils

Palmarosa Essence Oil

Lemon Essence Oil

Blending Glass Dram

Massage into skin

Joint Disorder Comfort - Temporomandibular

Supplies that you will need:

Bergamot Essence Oil

Helichrysum Essence Oil

Black Pepper Essence Oil

Juniper Berry Essence Oil

Frankincense Essence Oil

Chamomile (Roman) Essence Oil

Birch Essence Oil

Clove Bud Essence Oil

Eucalyptus Essence Oil

Mandarin Essence Oil

Lemon Essence Oil

Rosemary Essence Oil

Chamomile (German) Essence Oil

Peppermint Essence Oil

Ginger Essence Oil

Spearmint Essence Oil

Lavender Essence Oil

Laurel Essence Oil

Ylang Ylang Essence Oil

Rose Essence Oil

Blending Glass Dram

Massage into skin

Multiple Sclerosis

Supplies that you will need:

Cardamom Essence Oil

Bergamot Essence Oil

Grapefruit Essence Oil

Lemon Essence Oil

Melissa Essence Oil

Palmarosa Essence Oil

Pine Essence Oil

Ravensara Essence Oil

Rose Essence Oil

Sandalwood Essence Oil

Vetiver Essence Oil

Ylang Ylang Essence Oil

Helichrysum Essence Oil

Petitgrain Essence Oil

Juniper Berry Essence Oil

Frankincense Essence Oil

Chamomile (Roman) Essence Oil

Birch Essence Oil

Clove Bud Essence Oil

Neroli Essence Oil

Rosemary Essence Oil

Chamomile (German) Essence Oil

Peppermint Essence Oil

Clary Sage Essence Oil

Spearmint Essence Oil

Lavender Essence Oil

Laurel Essence Oil

Blending Glass Dram

Massage into skin

Migraines

Supplies that you will need:
Bergamot Essence Oil

Chamomile (Roman) Essence Oil

Neroli Essence Oil

Sweet Orange Essence Oil

Ginger Essence Oil
Peppermint Essence Oil
Lavender Essence Oil
Lemon Essence Oil
Grapefruit Essence Oil
Blending Glass Dram
St. John's Wort
Arnica
Massage into skin

Anxiety Calmer

Supplies that you will need:
Angelica Root Essence Oil
Cardamom Essence Oil
Cedarwood Essence Oil
Geranium Essence Oil
Juniper Berry Essence Oil
Frankincense Essence Oil
Chamomile (Roman) Essence Oil
Birch Essence Oil
Ginger Essence Oil
Jasmine Essence Oil
Mandarin Essence Oil
Grapefruit Essence Oil
Rose Essence Oil
Chamomile (German) Essence Oil

Peppermint Essence Oil
Clary Sage Essence Oil
Petitgrain Essence Oil
Myrrh Essence Oil
Sandalwood Essence Oil
Pine Essence Oil
Vetiver Essence Oil
Ylang Ylang Essence Oil
Melissa Essence Oil
Blending Glass Dram
Massage into skin

Neuralgia

Supplies that you will need:
Cardamom Essence Oil
Helichrysum Essence Oil
Lemongrass Essence Oil
Palmarosa Essence Oil
Melissa Essence Oil
Chamomile (Roman) Essence Oil
Birch Essence Oil
Clove Bud Essence Oil
Neroli Essence Oil
Sweet Marjoram Essence Oil
Pine Essence Oil
Ravensara Essence Oil

Chamomile (German) Essence Oil
Spearmint Essence Oil
Lavender Essence Oil
Laurel Essence Oil
Cinnamon Leaf Essence Oil
Vetiver Essence Oil
Blending Glass Dram
Massage into skin

Raynaud's Syndrome

Supplies that you will need:
Cardamom Essence Oil
Black Pepper Essence Oil
Petitgrain Essence Oil
Juniper Berry Essence Oil
Fennel Essence Oil
Eucalyptus Essence Oil
Rosemary Essence Oil
Peppermint Essence Oil
Clary Sage Essence Oil
Laurel Essence Oil
Cinnamon Leaf Essence Oil
Blending Glass Dram
Massage into skin

Hypertension

Supplies that you will need:

Angelica Root Essence Oil

Bergamot Essence Oil

Petitgrain Essence Oil

Patchouli Essence Oil

Frankincense Essence Oil

Chamomile (Roman) Essence Oil

Geranium Essence Oil

Sandalwood Essence Oil

Neroli Essence Oil

Sweet Marjoram Essence Oil

Sweet Orange Essence Oil

Grapefruit Essence Oil

Chamomile (German) Essence Oil

Vetiver Essence Oil

Clary Sage Essence Oil

Ylang Ylang Essence Oil

Lavender Essence Oil

Mandarin Essence Oil

Blending Glass Dram

Massage into skin

Hypotension

Supplies that you will need:

Black Pepper Essence Oil

Juniper Berry Essence Oil
Rosemary Essence Oil
Grapefruit Essence Oil
Peppermint Essence Oil
Ginger Essence Oil
Spearmint Essence Oil
Thyme Essence Oil
Blending Glass Dram
Massage into skin

Edema

Supplies that you will need:
Black Pepper Essence Oil
Juniper Berry Essence Oil
Rosemary Essence Oil
Grapefruit Essence Oil
Peppermint Essence Oil
Carrot Seed Essential Oil
Cypress Essence Oil
Geranium Essence Oil
Patchouli Essence Oil
Lemongrass Essence Oil
Lemon Essence Oil
Blending Glass Dram
Massage into skin

Infection

Supplies that you will need:

Cinnamon Leaf Essence Oil

Juniper Berry Essence Oil

Rosemary Essence Oil

Grapefruit Essence Oil

Eucalyptus Essence Oil

Geranium Essence Oil

Tea Tree Essence Oil

Lemongrass Essence Oil

Lemon Essence Oil

Ravensara Essence Oil

Thyme Essence Oil

Niaouli Essence Oil

Blending Glass Dram

Massage into skin

Cellulite Go Away

Supplies that you will need:

Cypress Essence Oil

Juniper Berry Essence Oil

Rosemary Essence Oil

Grapefruit Essence Oil

Eucalyptus Essence Oil

Ginger Essence Oil

Patchouli Essence Oil

Myrrh Essence Oil

Neroli Essence Oil

Blending Glass Dram

Massage into skin

Dysmenorrhea

Supplies that you will need:

Angelica Root Essence Oil

Birch Essence Oil

Lavender Essence Oil

Peppermint Essence Oil

Black Pepper Essence Oil

Cinnamon Leaf Essence Oil

Clary Sage Essence Oil

Patchouli Essence Oil

Vetiver Essence Oil

Ylang Ylang Essence Oil

Spearmint Essence Oil

Sweet Orange Essence Oil

Mandarin Essence Oil

Frankincense Essence Oil

Ginger Essence Oil

Helichrysum Essence Oil

Neroli Essence Oil

Geranium Essence Oil

Glass dram for blending

Massage onto skin

Amenorrhea

Supplies that you will need:
Angelica Root Essence Oil
Birch Essence Oil
Lavender Essence Oil
Peppermint Essence Oil
Black Pepper Essence Oil
Cinnamon Leaf Essence Oil
Clary Sage Essence Oil
Patchouli Essence Oil
Vetiver Essence Oil
Ylang Ylang Essence Oil
Spearmint Essence Oil
Sweet Orange Essence Oil
Mandarin Essence Oil
Frankincense Essence Oil
Ginger Essence Oil
Helichrysum Essence Oil
Neroli Essence Oil
Geranium Essence Oil
Chamomile (Roman) Essence Oil
Fennel Essence Oil
Glass dram for blending
Massage onto skin

Infertility

Supplies that you will need:

Bergamot Essence Oil

Jasmine Essence Oil

Melissa Essence Oil

Cardamom Essential Oil

Rose Essence Oil

Clary Sage Essence Oil

Chamomile (Roman) Essence Oil

Cypress Essence Oil

Neroli Essence Oil

Geranium Essence Oil

Fennel Essence Oil

Glass dram for blending

Massage onto skin

Blending Glass Dram

Irritable Bowel

Supplies that you will need:

Bergamot Essence Oil

Cardamom Essence Oil

Lavender Essence Oil

Peppermint Essence Oil

Black Pepper Essence Oil

Petitgrain Essence Oil

Clary Sage Essence Oil

Patchouli Essence Oil
Carrot Seed Essence Oil
Spearmint Essence Oil
Sweet Orange Essence Oil
Mandarin Essence Oil
Ginger Essence Oil
Neroli Essence Oil
Grapefruit Essence Oil
Juniper Berry Essence Oil
Glass dram for blending
Massage onto skin

Nausea

Supplies that you will need:
Cardamom Essence Oil
Lavender Essence Oil
Peppermint Essence Oil
Chamomile (Roman) Essence Oil
Carrot Seed Essence Oil
Spearmint Essence Oil
Mandarin Essence Oil
Ginger Essence Oil
Grapefruit Essence Oil
Rosemary Essence Oil
Glass dram for blending
Massage onto skin

Bronchitis

Supplies that you will need:

Cardamom Essence Oil

Lavender Essence Oil

Chamomile (German) Essence Oil

Cinnamon Leaf Essence Oil

Cedarwood Essence Oil

Peppermint Essence Oil

Clove Bud Essence Oil

Niaouli Essence Oil

Cyprus Essence Oil

Pine Essence Oil

Ravensara Essence Oil

Laurel Essence Oil

Fennel Essence Oil

Helichrysum Essence Oil

Ginger Essence Oil

Thyme Essence Oil

Frankincense Essence Oil

Lemon Essence Oil

Tea Tree Essence Oil

Glass dram for blending

Massage onto skin

Asthma

Supplies that you will need:

Cardamom Essence Oil

Bergamot Essence Oil

Chamomile (German) Essence Oil

Chamomile (Roman) Essence Oil

Cedarwood Essence Oil

Peppermint Essence Oil

Ylang-Ylang Essence Oil

Ravensara Essence Oil

Pine Essence Oil

Myrrh Essence Oil

Neroli Essence Oil

Eucalyptus Essence Oil

Patchouli Essence Oil

Petitgrain Essence Oil

Eucalyptus Essence Oil

Pine Essence Oil

Clary Sage Essence Oil

Rosemary Essence Oil

Glass dram for blending

Massage onto skin

Common Cold

Supplies that you will need:

Cardamom Essence Oil

Lavender Essence Oil

Chamomile (German) Essence Oil

Cinnamon Leaf Essence Oil

Cedarwood Essence Oil

Eucalyptus Essence Oil

Peppermint Essence Oil

Ginger Essence Oil

Niaouli Essence Oil

Cyprus Essence Oil

Pine Essence Oil

Ravensara Essence Oil

Laurel Essence Oil

Fennel Essence Oil

Helichrysum Essence Oil

Sandalwood Essence Oil

Thyme Essence Oil

Frankincense Essence Oil

Lemon Essence Oil

Tea Tree Essence Oil

Myrrh Essence Oil

Glass dram for blending

Massage onto skin

For Rooms Usage

Citrus Air Cleaner

Supplies that you will need:

Orange Essence Oil (10)

Grapefruit Essence Oil (50)

Patchouli Essence Oil (10)

Lime Essential Oil (50)

Purified Water (4 fl. oz.)

Use to purify or scent the room that you are in. This can be placed in a diffuser or a spray bottle for use when spraying the air.

Fruity Blend Air Refresher

Supplies that you will need:

Cedarwood Essence Oil (15)

Lemon Essence Oil (35)

Orange Essence Oil (50)

Grapefruit Essence Oil (20)

Purified Water (4 fl. oz.)

Use to purify or scent the room that you are in. This can be placed in a diffuser or a spray bottle for use when spraying the air.

Spring Blend

Supplies that you will need:

Clove Essence Oil (20)

Bergamot Essence Oil (50)

Mandarin Essence Oil (50)

Purified Water (4 fl. oz.)

Use to purify or scent the room that you are in. This can be placed in a diffuser or a spray bottle for use when spraying the air.

Summer Scent

Supplies that you will need:

Petitgrain Essence Oil (20)

Lemon Essence Oil (40)

Benzoin Essence Oil (20)

Lime Essence Oil (40)

Purified Water (4 fl. oz.)

Use to purify or scent the room that you are in. This can be placed in a diffuser or a spray bottle for use when spraying the air.

Flowers in Bloom

Supplies that you will need:

Rose Essence Oil (25)

Clove Essence Oil (20)

Orange Essence Oil (50)

Jasmine Essence Oil (10)

Cinnamon Essence Oil (15)

Purified Water (4 fl. oz.)

Use to purify or scent the room that you are in. This can be placed in a diffuser or a spray bottle for use when spraying the air.

Spring Flowers

Supplies that you will need:

Rose Essence Oil (75)

Clove Essence Oil (20)

Orange Essence Oil (25)

Purified Water (4 fl. oz.)

Use to purify or scent the room that you are in. This can be placed in a diffuser or a spray bottle for use when spraying the air.

Beautiful Bouquet

Supplies that you will need:

Rose Essence Oil (25)

Clove Essence Oil (20)

Geranium Essence Oil (35)

Peru Balsam Oil (15)

Bois De Rose Essence Oil (25)

Purified Water (4 fl. oz.)

Use to purify or scent the room that you are in. This can be placed in a diffuser or a spray bottle for use when spraying the air.

Wedding Bouquet

Supplies that you will need:

Ylang-Ylang Essence Oil (50)

Petitgrain Essence Oil (25)

Geranium Essence Oil (25)

Tolu Balsam Essence Oil (20)

Purified Water (4 fl. oz.)

Use to purify or scent the room that you are in. This can be placed in a diffuser or a spray bottle for use when spraying the air.

Walk in the Forest

Supplies that you will need:

Lavender Essence Oil (25)

Cedarwood Essence Oil (20)

Spruce Essence Oil (50)

Eucalyptus Essence Oil (25)

Purified Water (4 fl. oz.)

Use to purify or scent the room that you are in. This can be placed in a diffuser or a spray bottle for use when spraying the air.

Trees and Nature

Supplies that you will need:

Rosemary Essence Oil (30)

Lime Essence Oil (15)

Patchouli Essence Oil (15)

Spruce Essence Oil (30)

Myrtle Essence Oil (30)

Purified Water (4 fl. oz.)

Use to purify or scent the room that you are in. This can be placed in a diffuser or a spray bottle for use when spraying the air.

Nature's Best
Supplies that you will need:
Bois De Rose Essence Oil (30)

Eucalyptus Essence Oil (20)

Spearmint Essence Oil (30)

Spruce Essence Oil (40)

Purified Water (4 fl. oz.)

Use to purify or scent the room that you are in. This can be placed in a diffuser or a spray bottle for use when spraying the air.

Minty Fresh Air #1
Supplies that you will need:
Patchouli Essence Oil (10)

Petitgrain Essence Oil (20)

Peppermint Essence Oil (40)

Spearmint Essence Oil (10)

Caraway Essence Oil (40)

Purified Water (4 fl. oz.)

Use to purify or scent the room that you are in. This can be placed in a diffuser or a spray bottle for use when spraying the air.

Minty Fresh Air #2

Supplies that you will need:

Spearmint Essence Oil (40)

Rosemary Essence Oil (20)

Peppermint Essence Oil (10)

Benzoin Essence Oil (10)

Lime Essence Oil (10)

Lavender Essence Oil (30)

Purified Water (4 fl. oz.)

Use to purify or scent the room that you are in. This can be placed in a diffuser or a spray bottle for use when spraying the air.

Spicy Room Scent #1

Supplies that you will need:

Anise Essence Oil (10)

Cinnamon Essence Oil (20)

Ginger Essence Oil (20)

Clove Essence Oil (15)

Caraway Essence Oil (35)

Lime Essence Oil (10)

Purified Water (4 fl. oz.)

Use to purify or scent the room that you are in. This can be placed in a diffuser or a spray bottle for use when spraying the air.

Spicy Room Scent#2

Supplies that you will need:

Rosemary Essence Oil (30)

Cumin Essence Oil (20)

Allspice Essence Oil (25)

Coriander Essence Oil (25)

Clove Essence Oil (20)

Purified Water (4 fl. oz.)

Use to purify or scent the room that you are in. This can be placed in a diffuser or a spray bottle for use when spraying the air.

Romance Scent #1

Supplies that you will need:

Palmarosa Essence Oil (7)

Ylang-Ylang Essence Oil (7)

Bergamot Essence Oil (6)

Purified Water (4 fl. oz.)

Use to purify or scent the room that you are in. This can be placed in a diffuser or a spray bottle for use when spraying the air.

Romance Scent #2

Supplies that you will need:

Clary Sage Essence Oil (5)

Ylang-Ylang Essence Oil (5)

Black Pepper Essence Oil (5)

Clove Essence Oil (5)

Purified Water (4 fl. oz.)

Use to purify or scent the room that you are in. This can be placed in a diffuser or a spray bottle for use when spraying the air.

Romance Scent #3

Supplies that you will need:

Caraway Essence Oil (5)

Benzoin Essence Oil (5)

Patchouli Essence Oil (5)

Orange Essence Oil (5)

Purified Water (4 fl. oz.)

Use to purify or scent the room that you are in. This can be placed in a diffuser or a spray bottle for use when spraying the air.

Romance Scent #4

Supplies that you will need:

Sandalwood Essence Oil (7)

Orange Essence Oil (6)

Ylang-Ylang Essence Oil (7)

Purified Water (4 fl. oz.)

Use to purify or scent the room that you are in. This can be placed in a diffuser or a spray bottle for use when spraying the air.

Powders

Baby Powder #1

Supplies that you will need:

Cornstarch (2 tbsp.)

Bois De Rose (5)

Use on a baby for added freshness and an amazing smell.

Baby Powder #2

Supplies that you will need:

Cornstarch (2 tbsp.)

Lavender (5)

Use on a baby for added freshness and an amazing smell.

For Bath Usage

Easy Breathing Baths #1

Supplies that you will need:

Lavender (5)

Grapefruit (5)

Cajeput (5)

Carrier Oil (1tsp)

Blend together and place within your bath.

Easy Breathing Baths #2

Supplies that you will need:

Eucalyptus (4)

Petitgrain (1)

Anise (3)

Lemon (3)

Chamomile (4)

Carrier Oil (1 tsp.)

Blend together and place within your bath.

Easy Breathing Baths #3

Supplies that you will need:

Cajeput (5)

Peppermint (5)

Eucalyptus (5)

Carrier Oil (1tsp)

Blend together and place within your bath.

Easy Breathing Baths #4

Supplies that you will need:

Myrtle (4)

Grapefruit (1)

Rosemary (3)

Spruce (3)

Carrier Oil (1 tsp.)

Blend together and place within your bath.

Easy Breathing Baths #5

Supplies that you will need:

Myrtle (5)

Marjoram (3)

Lavender (5)

benzoin (2)

Carrier Oil (1 tsp.)

Blend together and place within your bath.

Easy Breathing Baths #6

Supplies that you will need:

Cajeput (5)

Spruce (5)

Lavender (5)

Carrier Oil (1 tsp.)

Blend together and place within your bath.

Calming Baths #1

Supplies that you will need:

Fennel (3)

Petitgrain (5)

Lavender (5)

Orange (2)

Carrier Oil (1 tsp.)

Blend together and place within your bath.

Calming Baths #2

Supplies that you will need:

Ylang-Ylang (5)

Petitgrain (5)

Orange (2)

Carrier Oil (1tsp)

Blend together and place within your bath.

Calming Baths #3

Supplies that you will need:

Geranium (5)

Lemon (5)

Sandalwood (5)

Carrier Oil (1 tsp.)

Blend together and place within your bath.

Calming Baths #4

Supplies that you will need:

Chamomile (5)

Peru Balsam (2)

Lemon (2)

Clary Sage (2)

Geranium (5)

Carrier Oil (1tsp)

Blend together and place within your bath.

Calming Baths #5

Supplies that you will need:

Mandarin (5)

Allspice (5)

Chamomile (5)

Carrier Oil (1 tsp.)

Blend together and place within your bath.

Calming Baths #6

Supplies that you will need:

Cypress (5)

Geranium (1)

Melissa (3)

Marjoram (3)

Lemon (3)

Carrier Oil (1 tsp.)

Blend together and place within your bath.

Setting the Mood While Bathing

Supplies that you will need:

Palmarosa (5)

Petitgrain (2)

Bois De Rose (5)

Grapefruit (3)

Carrier Oil (1 tsp.)

Blend together and place within your bath.

Introduction to Canine Section

I am so excited that you are on your way to understanding how to prepare oils for your dog by using the *Essential Oils for Dogs*. The following chapters will discuss how to use the oils best by using ways that will most benefit your pooch. First, let's consider how the oils came about in history.

The Ancient Egyptians were possibly one of the first cultures who realized that essential oils could be used for emotional benefits. Distillation methods were created by extracting oils from herbs, plants, and trees that were obtainable. These newly-found now ancient essential oils were used in daily activities including spiritual as well as medical—including embalming.

Cats are well known to have been embalmed by ancient Egyptians. However, many years later, it was discovered that millions of preserved dog mummies exist as well. Researchers found burial grounds in the catacombs south of Cairo filled with nearly 8 million mummified animals that were mostly dogs.

Ancient Romans, Greeks, Chinese, and various native cultures worldwide have utilized a distillation process of extracting the essential oils. Think back in time; there wasn't any canning or freeze-drying techniques available. With the use of this distillation, they could preserve the benefits of the various plants into a compact form without additional preservatives.

Progress rolled through the 1700s and 1800s when doctors, pharmacists, and other healers of that time prescribed essential oils to their patients many times. By the year of 1910, a French chemist and perfumer, [Rene Maurice Gattefosse, Ph.D.](), experienced a laboratory explosion, which resulted in the knowledge of lavender oil's ability to help heal burns.

I hope you enjoy each chapter and discover many new ways to help your dog. Every effort was made to ensure it is full of as much useful information as possible. If you are ever in doubt of the methods used, it would be best to receive professional assistance. The information provided in this book is for your general knowledge and education.

Before long, you will know which one of these oils will work best for your beloved dog. Many of the oils may already be in your inventory if you are already using essential oils. The most vital information to learn is that you must dilute the oils since they are toxic if too many oils are used in one product.

Chapter 1: Top Essential Oils for Your Dog

Essential oils can be used to treat infections, burns, viruses, depression, colds, and diseases of the immune system, and so much more in humans. It is absorbed through the cells, which will provide quick relief from many ailments to allow the body to begin healing quickly. They are powerful, yet mild so as not to harm the underlying cells while treating particular illnesses. Your pooch has never had it so good since, with time, people discovered the animals could also benefit from the oils at home.

Each of the oils in this list is considered safe for dogs according to favorite sources. However, it's always best to ask your veterinarian's opinion as well.

Angelica Root: *Angelica archangelica*: This oil can be used if your pooch suffers from irrational fears, especially if it's after an incident early in life. The oil is also good for animals who have on-going pain. It is antispasmodic, antifungal, expectorant, and much more.

Basil (linalool chemotype): *Ocimum basilicum* ct. linalool: It is known to be good for muscle aches, as an insect repellent, colds, coughs, and so much more.

Bergamot: *Citrus bergamia, Citrus aurantium*: This oil is a superb stress and anxiety reliever. You can also use it in a vaporizer, but be sure you have the proper dilution before applying to your dog's skin. Its pure form can burn the skin.

Cardamom: *Cardamomum*: This is an exceptional oil that provides many benefits for the respiratory and digestive system. Many experts believe cardamom oil can alter the mood of a dog that might be aggressive or anxious for different reasons. Diffuse the oil to create a calmer environment for your dog. It can also ease indigestion and calm an upset stomach.

Carrot Seed: *Daucus carota, Daucus carota* subspecies *sativa*: This essential oil is good for the skin. It has anti-inflammatory properties with moderate antibacterial effects. The oil is excellent for flaky, dry, or sensitive skin which is susceptible to infection. It can also stimulate tissue regeneration, so it is an excellent oil to use for scar healing.

Cedarwood (Atlas) or Himalaya: *Cedrus atlantica* or *deodara*: Your dog will love the calming and strengthening aura received from this great pest and flea repellent. It's also useful for kennel cough. Himalaya also stimulates circulation which is another alternative for your pooch if suffering from arthritis, stiffness, and back pain. It also helps clear up scruffy skin and dandruff, as it helps to stimulate hair growth. Other benefits include its ability to strengthen the kidney function, as a diuretic, lymphatic decongestant, and general tonic. It should help your pooch to lm down, especially for extreme timidity or shyness or nervous aggression.

Chamomile: Type 1: German Chamomile: *Matricaria recutita, Matricaria chamomilla, Chamomilla recutita* & **Type 2: Roman Chamomile**: *Chamaemelum nobile, Anthemis nobilis*: These oils soothe allergic reactions, burns, or skin irritations on your dog.

Clary Sage: *Salvia sclarea*: The clary sage oil is unique from common garden sage. It is gentle, sedating, and calming.

Eucalyptus: *Eucalyptus radiata*: Eucalyptus essential oil is an antiviral and anti-inflammatory. It is also an expectorant, so this oil is excellent to relieve chest congestion. This oil may help if your dog is suffering from an upper respiratory disease, such as bouts of kennel cough, and is coughing or having trouble breathing smoothly. Diluted properly, Eucalyptus essential oil is safe for dogs, both topically and for inhalation. Be sure NOT to let your dog ingest this oil, though. *Note*: Avoid using this oil with small dogs and puppies.

Frankincense: *Olibanum*: Frankincense is an exceptional 'all-around' oil since it isn't as potent versus numerous other essential oils. It can help to ease anxiety and to calm your pet. In some cases, it has helped with bouts of cancer as well as strengthening the immune system. Before using it, it's significant to consult with your vet to make sure this is vital for the issues plaguing your beloved pet. It is also safe for sheep, horses, goats, birds, and dogs.

Geranium: *Pelargonium graveolens, Pelargonium x asperum*: Geranium essential oil is safe and gentle for dogs. It is a robust antifungal oil and is suitable for skin irritations (primarily caused by yeast infections), as well as fungal ear infections in dogs. It is also effective in repelling ticks and is a must-have oil if you want to make your own tick-repelling oil blend for your dog.

Ginger: *Zingiber officinale*: Used in its diluted form, this oil is safe and non-irritating for dogs when used in small amounts. It is an excellent oil for dogs with motion sickness because of its anti-nausea elements. Ginger oil can also help with digestion and tummy upset. This oil also has pain-relieving properties. Used topically, it can help reduce pain in dogs with strains, sprains, dysplasia, or arthritis.

Helichrysum: *Helichrysum italicum*: This great oil is also sometimes called the "liquid Band-Aid" since it works as a super oil for skin regeneration and is also antibacterial. It reduces bleeding in accidents, helps repair nerves, and is beneficial for those who have cardiac disease or other heart-related issues.

Juniper Berry: *Juniperus communis*: This is a great fragrance oil and is also superb for other problems including shock, wound care, treatment of arthritis as well as some issues relating to the bladder. It is also safe for goats, horses, sheep, birds, and dogs.

Lavender: *Lavandula angustifolia, Lavender officinalis*: You may already realize that lavender is one of the gentler and more soothing of the essential oils. It is beneficial for fleabites and as a flea repellent. It can soothe the dog's state of mind as it soothes the skin. It is relaxing and mildly sedative as it steadies the heart, reduces anxiety, and may also help with hyperactivity. It is useful for bruises, grazes, or burns as an antiseptic to help wounds heal and prevent scarring. However, do not apply to deep wounds until you are positive that no infection is present. It is exceptional for hotspots and fungal infections. When purchasing lavender, make sure it is high quality and without unnecessary additives. It is also safe for horses, goats, sheep, birds, and dogs.

Lemon: *Citrus limon, Citrus limonum*: The use of lemon is known for clearing confusion and has many useful benefits. It is an excellent antiseptic, antifungal, an immune stimulant, antiviral, antidiabetic, anti-anemic, and anticoagulant. It also stimulates pancreatic function and antispasmodic for the stomach and breaks down excess bone deposits. Lemon has also been useful in the treatment of kidney stones or arthritis. In people, lemon helps increase the trust 'in self' and others which can also be helpful with dogs who have been relocated or have changed owners.

Mandarin (Green): *Citrus reticulata, Citrus nobilis*: This is undistilled and is a very sweet essential oil with very relaxing benefits. It is excellent for stress, anxiety, or for fearful situations your pup may encounter during the course of a day. Avoid red mandarin, which is not the same; use organic green mandarin only. This oil is pressed from the rind of the fruit.

Sweet Marjoram: *Origanum marjorana, Marjorana hortensis, Origanum dubium*: It has been noted to have antibacterial, antifungal, and antiseptic properties. It may also alleviate depression and nerve pain. These traits make it an excellent choice for skin allergy issues.

Myrrh: *Commiphora myrrha, Commiphora molmol*: Another great antioxidant for toothaches, dermatitis, acne, and sugar control. It is also safe for birds, horses, goats, and sheep.

Niaouli: *Melaleuca quinquinervia*: This is an exceptional oil for your dog with antibacterial properties to help eliminate allergies as well as its usefulness for its antihistamine elements.

Patchouli: *Pogostemon cablin, Pogostemon patchouli*: You can use this one if your dog has experienced trauma or abuse, and if he/she may also be sensitive to human touch. It is a grounding oil for a hyperactive dog.

Peppermint: *Mentha piperita*: Peppermint as an antiseptic, anti-inflammatory, and analgesic. Your pooch's airways can become clogged, and this is a great asset for those times as well as settling any digestive ailments. It is also safe for birds, goats, horses, and sheep.

Rose (Bulgarian, Damask): *Rosa damascene*: Rose oil is beneficial in many ways including the treatment of stress, eczema, depression, and symptoms of sexual dysfunction in dogs. Its extraction methods are usually expensive since it takes over 60,000 roses to create one ounce of essential oil.

Sandalwood: *Santalum spicatum, Santalum album*: India is where sandalwood has been used for religious ceremonies for centuries. The oil is derived from the matured sandalwood trees embedded in the oil's subtle, yet encompassing woody aroma. The tension will be relieved, stress senses calmed, and the skin hydration will be improved in your dog. You will be pleased to know that its effects are long-lasting.

Spearmint: *Mentha spicata, Mentha cardiaca, Mentha viridis, Mentha crispa*: Your veterinary can lend support to you if you choose to use spearmint oil for weight loss in your dog. In the short term, it can also address gastrointestinal problems such as colic and diarrhea if diluted in small amounts.

Sweet Orange: *Citrus x sinensis*: The sweet orange oil deters bugs and is also an excellent deodorizing agent. It is suitable for dogs with anxiety and depression. It can also stimulate a dog's appetite. If your dog is not eating (maybe due to stress or depression), diffusing this oil before mealtime may help. Since this oil has deodorizing and flea-repelling properties, it can also be added to your homemade doggie shampoo.

Thyme (linalool chemotype): *Thymus vulgaris* ct. linalool: There are many different chemotypes of thyme essential oil. The only chemotype that is mild and safe enough for dogs to use is thyme ct. linalool. This thyme oil has pain-relieving properties and can be added to a blend to help dogs with arthritis, rheumatism, or other joint pain. Additionally, it has powerful antibacterial, antifungal, and antiviral properties. It is an excellent choice for infections and other skin issues.

Valerian: *Valeriana officinalis*: If your dog suffers from separation or noise anxiety, the nerve-calming oil may just what is needed.

Vanilla: *Vanilla planifolia, Vanilla fragrans, Vanilla tahitensis*: Your pooch will love you for this one since it increases confidence and is an excellent choice for a training aid. It works well if your dog has repetitive negative behavior or separation anxiety.

Vetiver: *Vetiveria zizanoides, Phalaris zizanoides Andropogon muricatus, Chrysopogon zizanoides, Andropogon zizanoides*: If your dog is afraid of loud noises, vetiver oil might help lower the stress factor.

Yarrow: *Achillea Millefolium*: Purchasing the deep blue yarrow is a better anti-inflammatory than the green or pale blue version. Yarrow is a protective oil for wounds, stings, bites, allergies, and itchy skin. It can also be used to stop bleeding (such as one you would get from clipping your pup's toenails), as an anti-inflammatory for arthritis, sprains and pulls, ear infections, kidney infections, and physical or emotional trauma.

Ylang-Ylang: *Cananga odorata, Cananga odorata genuine*: The calming elements are beneficial for your dog and the oil is suitable for all skin types, even oily or inflamed skin. Drop a few drops into your dog's bath water for an effective treatment.

Other Oils for Dog

Cajeput: *Melaleuca cajuputi*
Caraway: *Carum carvi*
Cardamom: *Elatteria cardamomu*
Cinnamon Leaf: *Cinnamomum verum, Cinnamomum zeylanicum*
Cistus: *Cistus ladanifer, Cistus ladaniferus*
Citronella: *Cymbopogon winterianus, Cymbopogon nardus*
Coriander: *Coriandrum sativum*

Cypress: *Cupressus sempervirens*

Elemi: *Canarium luzonicum, Canarium vulgare*

Grapefruit: *Citrus paradise*

Lemongrass:*Cymbopogon flexuosus, Andropogon flexuosus, Cymbopogon citratus, Andropogon citratus*

Melissa: *Melissa officinalis*

Neroli: *Citrus x aurantium*

Nutmeg: *Myristica fragrans, Myristica moschata, Myristica aromatica, Myristica amboinensis*

Opopanax: *Commiphora erythraea, Commiphora guidottii*

Orange (Sweet, Blood): *Citrus sinensis, Citrus aurantium* var. sinensis

Palmarosa: *Cymbopogon martinii, Andropogon martinii* var. martinii, *Cymbopogon martinii* var motia

Petitgrain: *Citrus aurantium*

Plai: *Zingiber cassumunar, Zingiber montanum, Amomum montanum, Zingiber purpureum*

Rosalina: *Melaleuca ericifolia*

Rosemary: *Rosmarinus officinalis*

Spikenard: *Nardostachys grandiflora*

Tangerine: *Citrus reticulata, Citrus nobilis, Citrus tangeri*

Carrier Oils and Essential Oils Ratios

- *Avocado Oil* has the penetrative and excellent spreadability on the skin makes the avocado oils an ideal carrier oil. As you have guessed, it is extracted from the avocado which is rich in vitamin A, E, & D, lecithin, and essential fatty acids. It has effectively treated eczema and psoriasis in dogs. Another plus is that this oil is odorless.

- *Coconut Oil (cold-pressed)* is rich in lauric acid and is considered to be chosen as a high-quality oil for promoting healthy hair and skin. Coconut oil can also be added to your dog's food, but start in small amounts. Before adding, be sure to ask your vet. Coconut oil does so much more:

    a. *Improves Digestion*: It helps with coughing, reduces bad breath, nutrient absorption, and helps with colitis and inflammatory bowel syndrome.

    b. *Healthy Skin and Coat*: The oil minimizes dog odor, reduces allergic reactions, heals wounds, clears up eczema, relieves itchy skin, gives a shine to their coat, and more.

c. *It's a Superfood*: Coconut oil is an antifungal, antibacterial, antiviral, and aids in weight loss. It may also help to prevent infections and diseases, increases energy level, and much more.

- *Jojoba Oil* can also extend the life of the chosen essential oil product and leaves behind minimal residue. It is excellent for very oily or dry skin conditions. Jojoba oil is a bit nutty and has a longer shelf life than many of the other plant oils. Its texture is a sort of liquid wax extracted from jojoba seeds. It is odorless and excellent to use with lavender and peppermint. It can quickly help heal inflamed skin of the dogs created by psoriasis and eczema.

- *Olive Oil* is easily used for most preparations and works best with the extra virgin oil (EVOO) with more minerals and vitamins.

- *Sunflower Oil* is vitamin E rich and is an excellent source for body oils with its richness in fatty acids. It is known for moisturizing and soothing but also has a short shelf life. Be sure it is fresh; check the dates.

- *Sweet Almond Oil* is odorless and absorbs rapidly. It is excellent for massage and is also full of protein. The oil has been known for its penetrating, restructuring, and moisturizing benefits. It is a super remedy for inflammation, irritation, and itching brought on by dryness. The oil is extracted from nuts that are rich in minerals, proteins, vitamins as well as monounsaturated and polyunsaturated fatty acids.

Any of the vegetable, seed, or nut oils regularly used for cooking or food preparation can be used as carrier oil. However, be sure to search for unprocessed oils including those marked as organic or cold-pressed. Don't use the regular store oils which can contain petroleum residues and highly-refined solvents. The unprocessed oils are also the richest in proteins, minerals, and vitamins which help nourish the skin.

Other Carrier Oils

Arnica Oil works well for bruising and inflammation but should be avoided on broken skin.

Calendula Oil is a fabulous moisturizer and healer as a body oil for dry or damaged skin.

Canola Oil has a long shelf life. It is also light and odorless which is easily absorbed.

Castor Oil is a bit heavier than some oils, making it a superb choice as a moisturizer.

Corn Oil is loaded with minerals and vitamins and is used as medium weight oil.

Evening Primrose Oil is an antioxidant which will prolong the shelf life of the product.

Grapeseed Oil doesn't have a bold scent and dries quickly because of its high content of linoleic acid.

Hazelnut Oil is loaded with minerals, proteins, and vitamins.

Peanut Oil is rich in proteins and vitamins and is one of the most basic aromatherapy oils.

Safflower Oil is light to medium weight oil for softening your skin.

Sesame Oil has an SPF factor of 4 and is loaded with minerals, proteins, and Vitamin E which makes it a superb healer for many skin conditions.

Soy Oil is high in Vitamin E.

St. John's Wort Oil is excellent for inflammations of joints and muscles.

Vitamin E Oil also extends the shelf life of other carrier oils.

Walnut Oil is easily absorbed with medium weight and is suitable for your nervous system.

Wheat Germ Oil is good for burns and healing scars.

This list should keep you busy for a while!

Shopping Tips for the Carrier Oils

Search for premium quality carrier oils as you order and purchase your oils. You can buy them from health food stores, but they are a little more expensive. Check for lingering dust on the bottles which is a direct clue that the oil may not be fresh. Consider using suppliers/retailers that specialize in aromatherapy or natural skin care. Check the labels for additives or other oils that may be included in the bottle.

These are a few of those processes:

Shelf Life: As mentioned, the life of the chosen oil varies for each type. That is why it is vital to have a list ready to go before you purchase the ingredients including vitamin E, which is an antioxidant.

Nutrients: Many of the oils contain vitamins and fat-soluble minerals. Vitamin E, which acts as an antioxidant, will extend the life of the oil.

The Processing Method: Order oils that are cold-compressed, which is an indication that the oil was processed without applying excessive heat as it was derived from the fatty portions of particular plants. The high temperature could damage the nutrients in the carrier oil.

Organic Carrier Oils: As with any natural product, the cost is a bit more than others, but it should be certified.

Consider the Absorption or Feel of the Oil: The carrier oil should completely and quickly penetrate the skin. There won't be a sticky or oily residue after its application. Test a few drops in your hand.

The Color: No worries when it comes to the selection of an oil according to color. The only consideration that you will face is where more complex recipes are used when the color will matter. For your pet, it doesn't matter!

Aroma Expectations: You should consider a carrier oil that doesn't compete or conflict with the essential oil of choice.

The Price: As mentioned, the quality is paramount since you are preparing this for your dog. Your pet cannot tell how it feels when you apply the medications. You may also find a location where you can purchase the desired oils using special discounts or other promotions.

Important Information on the Bottle: Search for relevant information about the oils. You will find this on a brochure, the store's website, or printed on the bottle label. Notice that most of the oils listed have the information also. This is a list of the items:

- The common name of the oil
- Latin name of the oil
- How the oil was extracted
- Country of origin

- Method of cultivation (ex. cultivated, organic, wild-harvested, etc.)
- The words "100% pure essential oil" must be on the label.

How to Store the Carrier Oils

Proper storage is vital for the safety and integrity of the oils if you plan on using the same products for an extended period. You need to protect them from going rancid. Store them using tight lids and in dark-colored glass bottles. Place them in a cold and dimly lit area.

The carrier oils are generally packed into plastic bottles; it's not always poor quality, but an economical way of producing the oils. It merely saves the manufactures the additional expense of shipping the glass. Either way is acceptable for storing carrier oils, unlike the essential oils, which should be in a glass container. You can store most of the carrier oils in the fridge to increase the lifespan of some of the fragile oils.

Dangers of Rancidity

The shelf life of most carrier oil is from 0-15 months, depending on the type of oil, and how well it has been stored.

Borage oil, carrot oil, and evening primrose have a life of about 10-12 months, whereas grapeseed will last only 6-9 months. The carrier oils tend to become rancid quickly if not stored properly. It could take up to one year for that to occur, and most likely if you're an avid essential oil user, it will be gone before then. The essential oils don't go rancid.

Chapter 2: Preparation & Administering Pet Treatments

Signs Essential Oil Is Needed & What Method to Apply

Your dog will let you know when it's time to go shopping for essential oils. You may have noticed a bit of licking, sniffing, and localized digging. You need to decide how to administer the oils. These are some of the ways:

- *Orally*: Most dogs prefer to have the oils given orally if they suffer from a physical issue or if it's not too deeply-rooted. Be sure the oil is 100% pure and of a therapeutic grade. If your dog ingests the oil, only administer one drop and place it into an empty gel capsule in the food if they do not object.

    You can also take a clean toothpick and dip it into the oil. Use that to mix the oil into the food. It will quickly adhere to the chosen diet in amounts that can be easily handled by your dog.

- *Topical Application*: Your pooch might be more demanding and use a stamping of the feet or rubbing your body to indicate trouble spots. Just add a small amount to the area that your dog showed in his/her dog-like ways or apply it to the pads/toes, ears, and on the spine (leaving out the face).

- *Inhalation*: You can often put a dog into a deep sleep since it essentially sends the oils straight to the brain. The pros state that many treated dogs clear up emotional issues with just one sitting. Try adding one drop of the oil on the bed or the collar, or add it to a bottle and spritz the dog's coat. You can also add a few drops to your palm and let your pooch inhale its aroma.

Some essential oils may not cause an immediate effect and could take years to build up to levels that could harm your dog. That is why it's vital to know which ones are not allowed. You have to be sure the oil is pure. These are some of the ways to understand for sure:

- The bottle label should explicitly state it is 100% pure oil. If the contents are diluted, it will be noted on the bottle.

- Even though they are called 'oil', it doesn't mean they are oily to touch. Test it by rubbing a drop between your index and thumb. The essential oils should absorb directly into your skin and not stay on the surface.

- Don't skimp on the price because a little goes a long way. You are paying for its quality, not its quantity.

Vital First Steps for Administration of Essential Oils

- Choose the oil best chosen to treat your dog's ailments.
- Let your pooch smell each of the bottles with the lid on and undiluted.
- Pay close attention to your dog's reaction to the bottle's contents.
- It's vital to let your dog accept or refuse the oils you have chosen.

Safely Administer Essential Oils

Nature provides wild animals with minerals needed by eating plants. You have probably noticed your pooch grazing; it is instinct, which is scientifically known as 'Zoo-pharmacognosy'. As you allow your pet to sniff, you are letting that control for him/her to decide what will provide the most comfort and reduce the stress elements.

Provide 4 to 5 new aromas for a 'sniff-test' to determine which one is your pet's choice, but don't let your dog take off with the bottle. You will be able to tell because the dog will react!

Understand the Response

For the first phase of the introduction, you must be attentive to your dog and understand which direction your pet wants you to follow. As you offer the scent of the oil to your dog, watch the responses. To start, let your pooch see the bottle resting in your palm.

As your dog looks at it, if he/she begins to wag the tail or slurps with the tongue, you are a hit! However, if your pooch turns away with his/her head held low, that is a refusal. Just remain patient, if your pet stays in the room, it's time to prepare the recipe. Now, it's time to dilute the oil.

How to Dilute the Oil

The process is relatively simple once your dog has indicated which oil to use. Use 1 to 3 drops into one teaspoon of cold-pressed vegetable oil such as olive or sunflower oil. Offer the special oils separately and listen to the patient's response. Offer the oil once or twice each day until your dog doesn't seem to want it anymore. You can change the oils daily according to the responses. If the interest is peaked, try to dispense it two times a day or once if there's a disinterest. It shouldn't take more than three days to one week to see a remarkable change in the issues.

A word of caution: Always use the best quality essential oils and never forget to dilute them. Most of the smaller companies will cater to professional aromatherapists. Don't overuse the oils! They could cause skin irritation or liver failure.

Chapter 3: Marvelous Essential Oil Recipes to Pamper Your Pooch

This chapter is devoted to the medically-effective treatment options for your dog. Please experiment to discover a cure for your pooch's issues using one or a combination of the techniques. Once again, get a professional opinion—if in doubt. The recipes are prepared exclusively for dogs (not horses, cats, etc.).

Combat the Skin Issues

With dogs, skin conditions are preventable, but sometimes general issues can lead to more severe infections, rashes, and allergies. This segment will provide you with some of the choices you can use for specific problems.

- **Eczema**: Dermatitis is the redness and itching of your pup's skin. You may start noticing fur loss and skin infections as eczema progresses. Helichrysum is number one for the cure, but you can also use lavender, patchouli, and geranium.

- **Itching & Rashes**: Your dog might have reacted to fleas, a particular dog shampoo, or many other reasons. At any rate, lavender and peppermint oil are a superb treatment. Merely, apply it to the infected area.

- **Scarring**: If your dog got injured from scratching, you could eliminate some of the scarrings. Choose frankincense, rose, geranium, and lavender for some relief if scars develop.

- **Impetigo**: Younger dogs are more prone to become infected with impetigo, which is a bacterial skin condition that causes bumps on the dog's skin. They aren't acne but are filled with liquids which are vulnerable to ruptures. The discomfort or pain can be effectively treated using geranium oil and lavender.

- **Mange**: Mites are the culprit that can attach to hair follicles and the dog's skin to create a mild to severe skin infection. You may believe it is just a cluster of minuscule itchy bumps. However, you can apply peppermint oil to provide relief of the symptoms.

Combat Particular Illnesses

Fortunately, for your dog, you now have a plan to treat some of his/her issues using essential oils. These are just a few of them:

- **Diarrhea**: Your pooch may have food issues, infections, stress, or diarrhea including intestinal parasites. The symptoms become apparent with a liquid/loose stool. Try peppermint oil as a natural remedy by letting him/her inhale it. Do not apply it topically.

- **Vomiting**: Many elements can cause your dog to vomit. It could be caused by intestinal parasites, poisoning, heatstroke, or even kidney failure. Watch for the signs of abdominal heaving and drooling which is brought on by nausea. Include lavender, ginger, tarragon, and nutmeg oils for nausea. For vomiting, use nutmeg, peppermint, lavender, and patchouli oils for the best results.

- **Motion Sickness & Nausea**: Ease your pet's issues by using peppermint, chamomile, or sweet fennel.

- **Ear Infections**: Whether it's ear mites, allergies, or bacterial issues, you need to be aware of the symptoms. Be mindful of any shaking, tilting of the head, lack of balance, vigorous scratching, ear swelling, redness of the ear canal, a smelly odor in the ear, or redness in the ear canal. Clean the ear quickly to help clear the infections using bergamot, melrose, and lavender oils. Be sure to dilute using one of the vegetable oils. Use cotton swabs to clean the ears.

- **Coughing & Other Respiratory Problems**: Try using eucalyptus, myrrh, pine, or thyme oil for these issues for the best results.

Combat Behavioral Problems

Behavioral problems can be presented in the form of real stress for your pooch, which can cause depression, fear, or anxiety. You may notice your beloved dog beginning to show signs of aggression such as howling or barking at you. Try using sweet orange, jasmine, and rosemary oils to improve your dog's attitude. Experiment with valerian oil and roman chamomile oil using inhalation of vapors.

Recipes for Homemade Remedies for Your Pooch

Product 1: Doggy Shampoo

Product 2: Dry Skin Shampoo

Product 3: Anti-Itch Remedies

Product 4: Flea Control

Product 5: Dog Deodorant

Product 6: Calming Spray

Product 7: Ear Cleaner for Your Pooch

Product 8: Bath Water Oils

Product 9: Aging Dog Care

Product 10: Coconut Oil Antibiotic Cream

Product 11: Coconut Oil Paw Balm

Product 12: Arthritis Relief for the Pooch

Product 13: Dog Hyperactivity Spray

Product 14: Motion Sickness Spray

Product 15: Upset Tummy

Product 16: Sinus Infection Relief

Product 1: Doggy Shampoo

Option 1

Specific Use: To have a clean-smelling dog

What You Need:
- Water – 350 ml or 1.5 cup
- Castile soap – 1 tbsp
- Lavender essential oil – 2 drops
- Peppermint essential oil – 2 drops
- Rosemary essential oil – 2 drops
- Eucalyptus essential oil – 2 drops
- Bottle

How to Use:

1. Combine all of the components in a jar before adding to the shampoo container.
2. Be sure to shake the contents before using each time you bathe your dog.
3. Lather the dog from head to tail. Rinse well.

Option 2

What You Need:

- Liquid dish soap – 1 cup
- White vinegar – 1 cup
- Lavender essential oil – 2 drops
- Warm water – .5 cup

How to Use:

1. Combine all of the components and keep in a water bottle.
2. Massage into the fur and let it rest for a few minutes.
3. Rinse and dry your pup just as you usually do.

Option 3

What You Need:

- Lavender oil – 3 drops
- Peppermint oil – 3 drops
- Rosemary oil – 2 drops
- Eucalyptus oil – 3 drops
- Water – 250 ml

How to Use:

1. Blend all of the essential oil ingredients in a jar.
2. Mix with water and shake the bottle well.
3. Shampoo your dog.
4. Be sure to rinse thoroughly and towel dry.

Product 2: Dry Skin Shampoo

Specific Use: Flea & tick problems and dry skin

What You Need:

- Water – 1 cup
- Castile soap – 1 tsp.
- Vitamin E oil – .25 tsp.
- Roman chamomile oil – 2 drops
- Peppermint oil – 3 drops
- Purification oil – 2 drops
- Lavender oil – 3 drops
- Cedarwood oil – 1 drop
- Optional for fleas: Citronella oil – 2 drops

How to Use:

1. Combine all of the components in a glass jar. Mix well, and the shampoo is ready.
2. It may be slightly watery, but it is gentle and effective. As a flea shampoo, just add the citronella oil.

Product 3: Anti-Itch Remedies

Option 1: Dog Itches Be Gone

Specific Use: Dogs with itchy spots - Effective in decreasing itchiness and redness

What You Need:

- Carrier oil (Jojoba or Olive) – 5 oz.
- Lavender oil - 5 drops
- Vitamin E oil – 3 drops
- Roman chamomile oil – 5 drops
- Optional: Tea tree oil or Frankincense oil – 2-3 drops
- Also needed: 1 Glass dropper bottle

How to Use:

1. Combine all of the fixings into the bottle. Shake well.
2. Apply 2-3 drops on the spots as needed to help eliminate the itching spells.
3. They can also be used to reduce dry patches on the dog's skin.

Option 2: Coconut Oil Anti-Itch Cream
What You Need:

- Lavender essential oil – 10 drops
- Extra virgin organic coconut oil
- Lemon essential oil – 2 drops
- 1 glass bottle

How to Use:

1. Add the melted coconut oil into a small glass bottle.
2. Combine with the essential oils. Shake well.
3. Generally, an application using a topical massage will be sufficient. However, it's gentle enough to use as needed.

Product 4: Flea Control

Specific Use: For Collars

Two of the most common oils used for fleas are cedar and lavender oil.

What You Need:

- Water – 1-3 tbsp.
- Lavender or Cedar oil – 3-5 drops
- Dog collar or bandana
- Eye dropper

How to Use:

1. Use the water to dilute the oil and apply 5-10 drops of the solution to the dog's collar.
2. Reapply the oil about once each week.

Specific Use: Fleas Around The Tail

What You Need:

- Cedar or Lavender oil – 1-2 drops

- Olive oil – 1 tbsp.

How to Use:

1. Shake the bottle well and place on the base of the dog's tail.

Specific Use: Flea Spray

What You Need:

- White or Apple cider vinegar – 1 cup or 50/50 combo
- Fresh water – 1 quart
- Lavender oil or Cedar oil – 2-3 drops
- Spray bottle

How to Use:

1. Combine all of the components in the spray bottle and shake well.
2. Mist the dog with the spray, avoiding the nose, ears, and eyes.
3. Be sure you take a cloth with the mixture and apply behind the ears and around the entire neck area.
4. Give the pet's bedding a misting during the process.

Product 5: Dog Deodorant

Specific Use: Help make your dog smell terrific!

What You Need:

- Spray bottle
- Peppermint oil – 6 drops
- Lavender oil – 10 drops
- Sweet orange oil – 6 drops
- Eucalyptus oil – 3 drops
- Purified water – 8 oz.

How to Use:

1. Mix all of the oils and water and shake well.
2. Be sure you cover your dog's face and eyes.
3. Spray the coat thoroughly to remove the 'bad doggie' odors.
4. Tip: Keep this handy for those rainy-day dog aromas! Spray the house with the homemade household spray (see the recipe).

Product 6: Calming Spray

Specific Use: If your pooch has a hard time settling down, try some of this spray!

What You Need:

- Water – 1.5 cups
- Roman chamomile essential oil – 5-10 drops
- Lavender essential oil – 5-10 drops
- Spray bottle

How to Use:

1. Mix all of the ingredients thoroughly.
2. Pour into the bottle and shake the contents before using.
3. Spray a misting over the dog as needed.

Product 7: Ear Cleaner For Your Pooch

Specific Use: Improve your dog's ear health

What You Need:

- Geranium oil – 5 drops
- Lavender oil – 5 drops
- Melaleuca oil – 5 drops
- Coconut oil – 1 tbsp.

How to Use:

1. Combine all of the ingredients.
2. Clean your dog's ears with a natural cleaner.
3. Gently use a Q-tip to run the mixture into the ears, making sure not to immerse it further than you can see the tip.
4. Clean with the oil mixture twice each day until it clears.

Product 8: Bath Water Oils

Add the chosen essential oil to the water and disperse it evenly before your pooch jump into the mixture. The aromatic molecules in the oil can penetrate your dog's skins as he/she breathes the aromas. These are some of the special ones for a quick splash:

- **Lavender Oil**: Supports irritated and damaged skin quicker than the spray bottle lavender sprays.

- **Jasmine Oil**: An excellent uplifting aroma for the pooch.

- **Vetiver Oil**: A great moisturizer can help work miracles.

- **Rose Oil**: Uplifts your pooch's mood and lower the anxiety levels as needed.

Product 9: Aging Dog Care

Specific Use: Remedy for different aches and pains for older dogs

What You Need:

- Peppermint oil – 3 drops
- Carrier oil – 3 tsp.
- Lavender oil – 3 drops
- Balsam fir oil – 2 drops
- Copaiba oil – 2 drops

How to Use:

1. Combine all of the oils and mix well.
2. This can also be applied as an ointment to the pet's food pad for quicker absorption.

Product 10: Coconut Oil Antibiotic Cream

Specific Use: Remedy for any areas that need a special healing cream

What You Need:

- Oregano essential oil – 12 drops
- Coconut oil – 4 tbsp.

How to Use:

1. Melt the coconut oil and add it to a bottle or glass jar.
2. Add the orange oil and mix with a spoon.
3. Massage onto your dog's skin.

Product 11: Coconut Oil Paw Balm

Specific Use: Remedy for any healing sore paws

What You Need:

- Natural beeswax – 8 tbsp.
- Extra virgin organic coconut oil
- Olive essential oil – 4 tbsp.
- Shea butter – 2 tbsp.
- 2 storage tins or jars
- 1 small pot

How to Use:

1. Add all of the fixings to a small pot using the low-heat setting on the stovetop.
2. Stir until blended and melted. Pour into the jars/tins. Let the mixture cool and harden.
3. Cap and label the balm "For External Use Only", so no one thinks it is non-toxic for consumption.
4. A wide-mouth container is best for storage so you can rub your dog's paw over the surface for application.
5. Be sure to store the balm away from sunlight and direct heat.

Product 12: Arthritis Relief for the Pooch

Option 1:

What You Need:

- Ginger essential oil – 8 drops
- Sweet almond or Jojoba carrier oil – 4 oz.
- Lavender essential oil – 6 drops
- Lemon essential oil – 8 drops

How to Use:

1. Apply topically by placing the drops in your hands.
2. Massage the sore joints for your pooch.
3. Add 2-3 drops inside the tips of the dog's ears.

Option 2:

What You Need:

- Valerian essential oil – 7 drops
- Jojoba or Sweet almond carrier oil – 4 oz. or 120 ml
- Helichrysum essential oil – 8 drops
- Ginger essential oil – 5 drops

- Peppermint essential oil – 4 drops

How to Use:

1. Thoroughly apply the medicine topically on your dog by rubbing 2-3 drops of the oil in your hands.
2. Massage the painful or sore joint of your dog.
3. Add a couple of drops inside of the ear tips.

Product 13: Dog Hyperactivity Spray

What You Need:

- Jojoba, Olive, or Sweet Almond carrier oil – 4 oz.
- Bergamot oil – 3 drops
- Lavender oil – 6 drops
- Roman chamomile oil – 5 drops
- Valerian oil – 6 drops
- Sweet marjoram oil – 4 drops

How to Use:

1. You can use this one topically or aromatically.
2. Spray the mixture onto your dog's coat each day, making sure you avoid his/her face area.
3. Also, spray the contents on the bedding and around the doorways to eliminate the invasion of pests.

Product 14: Motion Sickness Spray

What You Need:

- Peppermint oil – 10 drops
- Ginger oil – 14 drops
- Sweet almond, Jojoba, or Olive carrier oil – 120 ml or 4 oz.

How to Use:

1. You can apply to your dog either aromatically or topically.
2. Avoid the eyes and spray under the armpit, his belly, and the tip of his/her ears.

Product 15: Upset Tummy

What You Need:

- Peppermint essential oil – 2-3 drops
- Coconut or Olive carrier oil – 5-6 drops

How to Use:

Mix all of the components and apply the blend to your dog's stomach.

Product 16: Sinus Infection Relief

What You Need:

- Sweet almond oil – 15 ml
- Ravensare essential oil – 5 drops
- Eucalyptus essential oil – 5 drops
- Myrrh essential oil – 5 drops

How to Use:

1. Mix all of the fixings thoroughly.
2. Apply topically by applying a few drops onto the dog's chest and neck.

Chapter 4: Precautions Using Essential Oils

As mentioned, some oils are okay for horses and dogs, while smaller animals including rabbits and birds cannot tolerate them primarily because of the smaller bodies. Please acknowledge all of the products listed in this segment, beginning with the 'maybe' not-so-favorite Tea Tree:

Tea Tree: *Melaleuca alternifolia*: Documentation has been provided that indicates tea tree oil might have more harmful effects versus the benefits for your dog. Follow the instructions provided by a veterinarian (not hearsay) if you choose to use the oil. If unsure, you should ask for another form of treatment. If you decide to start the procedure, remember that the essential oils must always be diluted.

Wintergreen: *Gaultheria procumbens*: The oil is derived from the eastern teaberry oil of wintergreen containing aspirin (methyl salicylates). For humans, it's generally used topically for pain including achy muscles. However, dogs can show signs of 'aspirin toxicity' which may be displayed with bouts of vomiting due to severe gastrointestinal upset. If your dog becomes 'toxic,' seek vet care for support.

European Pennyroyal: *Mentha pulegium*: This old folk medicine recipe, also known as squaw mint, is used as an insect repellent. The toxicity with pennyroyal can cause liver failure or hepatic necrosis. Symptoms can consist of diarrhea or vomiting which can be indications of the deadly poisoning effects.

Pine: These are derived from the Scots Pine (*Pinus sylvestris*) located in Europe. Pine oils are incorporated in cleaning products as a disinfectant and deodorizer. The touted benefits of pine oil include its ability to help with tenderness and pain in sore joints, aid in decreasing swelling, increasing circulation, and muscles. Unfortunately, in dogs, with dermal or oral exposure can have gastrointestinal irritation, weakness, drooling, and vomiting that may be bloody. Emergency care is probably necessary if these signs are present.

Other Oils to Never Use on Your Dog

Anise (*Pimpinella anisum*)
Birch (*Betula*)
Bitter Almond (*Prunus dulcis*)
Boldo (*Peumus boldus*)
Calamus (*Acorus calamus*)

Camphor (*Cinnamomum camphora*)

Cassia (*Cassia fistula*)

Chenopodium (*Chenopodium album*)

Cloves (*Syzygium aromaticum*)

Garlic (*Allium sativum*)

Goosefoot (*Chenopodium murale*)

Horseradish (*Armoracia rusticana*)

Hyssop (*Hyssopus* sp. with the exception of Decumbens)

Juniper (*Juniperus* sp. with the exception of Juniper Berry)

Mugwort (*Artemisia vulgaris*)

Mustard (*Brassica juncea*)

Red or White Thyme (*Thymus vulgaris*)

Rue (*Ruta graveolens*)

Santolina (*Santolina chamaecyparissus*)

Sassafras (*Sassafras albidum*)

Savory (*Satureja*)

Tansy (*Tanacetum vulgare*)

Terebinth (*Pistacia palaestina*)

Thuja (*Thuja occidentalis*)

Wormwood (*Artemisia absinthium*)

What to Do If Poisoning Is Suspected

Remember the basics:

- Do not add the essential oils to your dog's drinking water or food unless diluted (unless vet approved).
- Use hydrosols with puppies under ten weeks of age—not essential oils.

Since the viscosity of oils and aspiration pneumonia are a risk factor if the dogs ingest the oil and get it in their lungs, the irritation can cause problems to the gastrointestinal tract. It will cause the oil to be aspirated when it is vomited. Immediate veterinary care is needed with most of these exposures.

Be a fabulous dog owner and learn that prevention is the best medicine in limiting essential oil toxicities. Once again, it is highly recommended to discuss the use of essential oils with your veterinarian before using. If they do not have experience with essential oils, they should be able to refer you to someone in the veterinary profession who can give you the information needed for safe use of essential oils.

Remember, accidents do happen, so keep the _ASPCA Animal Poison Control Center_ hotline on a notepad where it can be easily located. Call anytime at **888-426-4435**.

Checkpoints and Safety Tips

Some dogs are more sensitive than others, so as you get your oils together, be sure to avoid the following chemicals:

- Benzalkonium chloride
- Benzethonium chloride
- Dioxins
- Diaminobenzene
- Methicone
- Diethanolamine
- Petrolatum
- Propylene glycol
- Sodium lauryl sulphate
- Sodium hydroxide

How to React If Your Dog Is Allergic to an Essential Oil

- Wash off the oil if you applied it topically.

- Make sure they don't come in contact with the oil again.

- Discontinue use of the oil they are allergic to.

- Take them to the vet if need be.

Safety Tips for Using Essential Oils on Your Dogs

- Start by using essential oils that are highly diluted on dogs.
- Avoid contact with the snout, eyes, anal glands, and genitals.
- Never expose a dog to an undiluted form of any essential oil.
- Check with your vet before giving internally to go over possible side effects.
- Avoid giving oils internally if you're worried about potency. You must be sure of the exact amount is needed according to your dog's weight.
- Steer clear of oils that dogs are more sensitive to.

How to Remove the Oil If It Causes a Burning Sensation

Your dog's skin may be too sensitive for some of the oils you choose to apply. Try not to panic. Don't use soap and water to attempt washing it away because that will only make the oils spread. Instead, liberally apply some vegetable oil to dilute the essential oil overdose. Almost immediately, once the oils blend together, the discomfort is removed. Apply as much as needed.

Remember the logic of it all: with dogs and essential oils, generally, 'less is more.' Just remember you cannot use the human application amounts with dogs or any other animal.

Chapter 5: Clean-Up Time for Your Pooch

Once, you have the knack of making oils for your dog, why not go 'natural' and prepare some cleaners that will be safer four his/her living spaces.

All-Purpose Cleaner or Window Cleaner

Lemon Household Cleaner

Natural Toilet Bowl Scrubber

The Vacuum Cleaner

Delightful Scents Air Freshener Sprays

Gel Air Fresheners

All-Purpose Cleaner Or Window Cleaner

Dogs love to sniff, and windows are no exception!

What You Need:

- Water and white or apple cider vinegar – Equal parts
- Orange or Lemon essential oil – 10-15 drops
- 1 spray bottle

How to Use:

1. Combine the products in a spray bottle.
2. Shake well and use to remove the grime or just make the windows sparkle.

Lemon Household Cleaner

What You Need:

- Water – 8 oz.
- Distilled white vinegar – 4 oz.
- Tea tree oil – 15 drops
- Lemon essential oil – 15 drops
- Also needed: Glass cleaning spray bottle

How to Use:

1. Fill the bottle with all the ingredients and mix.
2. Shake the contents before each cleaning spray.
3. *Tip:* It is advisable to use a glass container when possible. The citrus essential oils are highly concentrated and have acidic properties. Sometimes, it is best to store the products in glass for this reason.

Natural Toilet Bowl Scrubber

No matter how many times, you close the toilet bowl lid, your pooch will find a way to drink out of it. Try these combinations:

What You Need:

- Vinegar – 1 cup
- Borax – .75 cup
- Tea tree essential oil – .5 tsp.
- Lemon essential oil – 5 drops

How to Use:

1. Combine all of the ingredients in a medium glass container.
2. Use .25 to .5 cup into the toilet bowl.
3. Let it sit for several minutes. Use a brush to remove the stains.
4. *For a spray:* You can also make it a bit thinner to use as a spray.
5. *For a scrub:* Add .25 cup of baking soda to the mix and use gloves to scrub the toilet.

The Vacuum Cleaner

How to Use:

1. Add 2 to 3 drops of your favorite clean-smelling aroma to the bag or filter of your vacuum cleaner.
2. Keep in mind that you can use your dog's favorite scent. After all, you can both enjoy a little serenity.

Delightful Scents Air Freshener Sprays

What You Need:

- Filtered water – 6 tbsp.
- Vodka – 1 tbsp.
- Essential oil of choice: citrus, peppermint, jasmine, or lavender – 10-40 drops

How to Use:

1. Place the alcohol and oils in a small spray bottle.
2. Shake well and add the water.
3. Shake before you spritz whenever you want to be energized.

Here are a few more versions using another method for sprays:

Lavender Linen: 2 oz. size

- Witch hazel oil – 1 tsp.
- Distilled water – almost 2 oz.
- Lavender oil – 15-20 drops

- Dark spray bottle – 2 oz.

Energy Boost: 3 oz. size

- Lemon oil – 20 drops
- Eucalyptus oil – 8 drops
- Peppermint oil – 2 drops
- Cinnamon oil – 2 drops

Fresh Floral: 3 oz. size

- Rosemary oil – 6 drops
- Frankincense oil – 4 drops
- Juniper oil – 8 drops
- Jasmine oil – 6 drops

Sweet Citrus: 3 oz. size

- Lavender oil – 10 drops
- Sweet orange oil – 8 drops
- Vanilla oil – 4 drops
- Bergamot oil - drops

How to Use:

1. Add the lavender oil, witch hazel oil, and distilled water.
2. Spray your linens and pillows for a tantalizing effect.

Gel Air Fresheners

This is so simple to prepare. Lavender and lemon are excellent for serenity (merely prepare with your dog's favorite.).

What You Need:

- Knox Gelatin – 1 packet
- Water – .75 cup
- Vodka – .25 cup
- Essential oil of your choice – 15 drops

- Food coloring – 1-2 drops

How to Use:

1. Bring the water to a boil in a small pan and add the gelatin pack.
2. Stir until dissolved. Allow it to cool at room temperature.
3. Pour into a small jar. Add the oils, vodka, coloring, and any decorative items. Stir and place in the refrigerator until set.
4. You can be creative by adding decorations in the gel. You can also add a wick to the bottom of the glass and make a gel candle.
5. *Note:* As the aroma fades, you can add a few more drops.

Shelf Life of Homemade Essential Oil Products

Most essential oils will last from 1 to 3 years if they are stored in a glass jar or vial. A cobalt or amber color is best.

The average shelf life of the vegetable oil is approximately 6 months. However, it would need to be refrigerated in a closed container. It is recommended to write the purchase or prepared date on the bottle. The shelf life can be extended each item you add an antioxidant to your essential oil blends. Citrus oil only lasts from 6 months to 1 year as well.

Prevent cross-contamination by using a separate glass dropper for each of the oils. It will also make the oils more diluted if you accidentally mix the aromas. Unless you use the oil frequently, it is best to store it with its original top. The rubber dropper could pucker if it is too tight or loose.

Chapter 6: Specials For Mom & Dad

Now, it is time for you to have some special times with essential oils. After a hard day of hiking with your pooch, it is time to relax!

Massage Oils

- **Uplifting Mental Clarity: Warm Spice Blends**

For these blends, use almond, coconut, or jojoba as the carrier oil.

Cardamom Oil is used to invigorate your mind and body to ease nervous tension.

Cinnamon Bark Oil is used as a potent/natural stimulant. It is also antimicrobial and helps to promote digestive health. Apply 5 to 6 drops of the base - dry/warm herbal spice.

Coriander Seed Oil soothes inflammation, stimulates the senses, and aids in digestion. Apply 3 to 4 drops of the middle - spicy/woody/fruity aroma.

Sweet Orange Oil displays an uplifting and cleansing aroma as a top note: fruity/citrusy spice. Apply 14 to 16 drops for a luxurious massage.

- **Sensuality and Emotional Well-Being: The Citrus Flower Blend**

For these blends, use olive, grapeseed, or olive as the carrier oil.

Bergamot Oil elevates your mood and relieves tension with 12 to 14 drops of oil. The group is top note: spicy, floral, and citrus aromas.

Clary Sage Oil will naturally elevate your mood and soothe the tension with the middle - musky, floral, bitter-sweet aroma. Use 2 to 3 drops of oil for the massage.

Grapefruit Oil is a secondary top note oil - tangy, fresh, and citrus tones to promote detoxification and help improve your skin health. Use 2 to 3 drops of oil for best results.

Jasmine Oil is of the middle - intensely floral, warm, and rich oil category. You will stimulate your senses and warm your body. Use only 2 to 3 drops.

Vanilla Oil is a superb mood enhancer. Only 4 to 5 drops are necessary for the base: creamy floral, sweet, and rich.

Ylang-Ylang is known as relaxing and mood-elevating oil with the sweet, rich, floral base. A mere 2 to 3 drops will work the magic.

- **Relax Your Mind and Body: Sweet Dreams Massage**

For these blends, use grapeseed as the carrier oil:

Chinese Rose is the middle category with its spicy, sweet, floral oil will add depth to the aroma with just 2 to 3 drops.

Lavender Oil is the middle category with its floral, sweet aromas as a powerful detoxifier. With 12 to 14 drops of oil, you will receive its anti-inflammatory features for a great night of sleep.

Sandalwood Oil has light balsam and woody notes. Sandalwood is a decongestant. Its soothing anti-inflammatory features are flowing after 3 to 4 drops are applied to your skin.

Valerian Oil sends anxiety away with this natural sleep aid from the base category of woody, musky, and warm oil. Use 6 to 7 drops for an ultimate sleep.

Bay Oil

An intense fragrance similar to clove oil is present with this unique oil. You can use it as a massage oil or add it to a vaporizer or burner. Small amounts can produce a stimulant, whereas a more substantial amount of oil can create a sedative effect. It is useful for these:

Depression

What to Use:

- Jojoba oil – 1 tbsp.
- Bay oil – 2 drops
- Black pepper oil – 4 drops
- Bergamot oil – 4 drops

Relaxation

What to Use:

- Bay oil – 10 drops
- Clove oil – 1 drop
- Sweet orange oil – 2-3 drops
- Almond oil for the carrier oil

Stress Reduction

A 2013 research study discovered sniffing chamomile, lavender, and neroli is beneficial in reducing stress and anxiety.

What to Use:

- Lavender – 3 drops
- Marjoram – 3 drops
- Unscented lotion – 15 ml

How to Use:

Blend the mixture to ease your tightened muscles and relax your tense mind.

As a Final Summary

Even though essential oils are useful in healing, they are mighty and can also carry a wide range of contrary effects. You need to be sure that you safely and accurately measure the oils. The most significant issue involved using essential oils is that they might encompass pollutants that can cause more pressing issues. For this purpose, you should use only therapeutic grade oils purchased from reliable companies and confirm the quality of oils before consuming or using them on your dog.

Your dog has a sensitive sense of smell. If your dog doesn't like an oil—definitely—don't enforce its use. Since animals metabolize and react differently to essential oils, it is critical to know about species-specific differences before using oils. People overusing oils is a common issue.

To reduce the chances of sensitivity and organ toxicity, you should generally use oil for no more than two weeks and then provide a rest period. Under certain circumstances, you could use them for more extended periods, but this is something best left to those trained in the use of oils.

Conclusion

Now that you have made it to the end of this *Essential Oil and Aromatherapy* book, I hope you have a wider understanding of the uses of Essential Oils. Essential Oils have been around for centuries and with so much documented information about Essential Oils, it's no wonder you are interested in learning more.

Essential oils can be used for some many different medicinal and environmental purposes. That is why several cultures have been using Essential Oils since prior to 1500 B.C.

This book is just a small portion of what you can expect when learning about Essential oils. There is so much more that you could learn. By starting with this book, you are building a good foundation to get started with using Essential Oils and helping your family be healthier.

Essence oils are a wonderful way to utilize alternative medical remedies without all the pressure that medical doctors and medicine adds to your life. Many people have found that by using essential oils, they are able to get the relief they needed but was not able to find through modern medicine. Many doctors are now turning to alternative remedies for those patients that have struggled with healing. They have seen the benefits of essential oils and know that there is a lot more to learn about plant essentials.

An aromatherapist is someone that utilizes essential oils to help alleviate and heal your mind, body, and soul. I have included enough recipes to help you have a clear understanding of what types of recipes you can make with Essential Oils. Although blending is a technique it is not always necessary to blend more than one oil. You can sometimes use just one oil that is blended with a carrier oil for your needs. There are a few oils that are in a lower concentration level which can be used without a carrier oil.

I also hope that you are dedicated to utilizing this book and all the materials within it to advance your weight loss efforts. With all the recipes within this book, you should have no reason to still be looking for a way to increase the efforts that you have applied to weight loss and to advance your reduction in pounds. I am sure that you are.

If you have found this book helpful I hope that you leave a wonderful review so that others will find it just as helpful.

Canine Section's Conclusion

I hope you have enjoyed learning about how to use *Essential Oils for Dogs*. Let's hope it was informative and provided you with all of the information you need to achieve your goals working with your pooch for relaxation and better health.

The next step is to decide which of the oils will be the most beneficial for your beloved dog. Essential oils have tons of benefits for dogs, and they are truly remarkable! You now have all of the information to provide a much happier life for your pooch, and you have already made the biggest step when you added this book to your files. Try using the selected oils for two weeks and take a break. You will be able to decide whether the oils are doing the job.

You now have the tools at your fingertips that are needed to give your pet all the essential oils have to offer. Finally, if you find this book useful in any way, a review on Amazon is always appreciated!

CPSIA information can be obtained
at www.ICGtesting.com
Printed in the USA
LVHW021052240920
666994LV00002B/273